MENOPAUSE, SISTERHOOD, AND TENNIS

T0273438

MENOPAUSE, SISTERHOOD, AND TENNIS

A MIRACULOUS JOURNEY THROUGH "THE CHANGE"

ALICE WILSON-FRIED

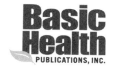

Basic Health
PUBLICATIONS, INC.

The information contained in this book is based upon the research and personal and professional experiences of the author. It is not intended as a substitute for consulting with your physician or other healthcare provider. Any attempt to diagnose and treat an illness should be done under the direction of a healthcare professional.

The publisher does not advocate the use of any particular healthcare protocol but believes the information in this book should be available to the public. The publisher and author are not responsible for any adverse effects or consequences resulting from the use of the suggestions, preparations, or procedures discussed in this book. Should the reader have any questions concerning the appropriateness of any procedures or preparation mentioned, the author and the publisher strongly suggest consulting a professional healthcare advisor.

BASIC HEALTH PUBLICATIONS, INC.
8200 Boulevard East • North Bergen, NJ 07047 • 1-201-868-8336

Library of Congress Cataloging-in-Publication Data

Wilson-Fried, Alice.
    Menopause, sisterhood, and tennis: a miraculous journey through "the change" / Alice Wilson-Fried.
        p. cm.
Includes bibliographical references and index.
    ISBN 1-59120-076-8
    1. Wilson-Fried, Alice, 1948–   Health.   2. Menopause—Biography.
I. Title.

    RG186.W53   2003
    362.1'98175'0092—dc21

                                    2003010430

Editor: Nancy Ringer
Typesetter/Book design: Gary A. Rosenberg
Cover design: Mike Stromberg

Printed in the United States of America

10   9   8   7   6   5   4   3   2   1

Contents

*To my youngest brother, Lloyd,
a die-hard sports enthusiast,
who passed away before he saw
what he called "a miracle"—
me playing tennis.*

Acknowledgments

My sincere thanks to my husband, Frank, whose faith in me keeps me going; to Fay Greenfield and Anne Fox, for their red editing pencils; to my sisterfriend, Jewel Bleckinger, for her encouragement; to Sam Gelfman, for showing me the way to my agent, Al Zuckerman, and to Al himself, who didn't give up on me despite the rejections; to my kids and grandkids, for empowering me with their unconditional love and filling me with pride; and to my tennis sisterfriends, who simply spice up my life.

Introduction

My inners, as my grandmother would say, were in turmoil. I had the energy of a gnat, couldn't think, and couldn't sleep. I craved and ate so much sweet and starchy food that my thyroid stopped metabolizing. I cried for no reason. I went into temper tantrums without provocation. Hell, I couldn't reason my way out a confrontation with my two-year-old grandchild.

My husband, Frank, a former tennis player and avid fan of the game, suggested that I take up the sport. He argued that the game would get me out and about, put me in touch with other people, particularly women my own age. Tennis, he told me, might give me the physical outlet I needed to put some distance between my brain and the inevitable hormonal changes I was experiencing.

"Me, play tennis?" I responded. Understand, I would have flunked high-school physical education if not for the written exam and the extra points awarded for simply wearing the gym suit. You see, I'm the crossword-puzzle type, the bookworm. A *Matlock* and *In the Heat of the Night* groupie. If computers had been around when I was a kid, I would have been the classic nerd.

Besides, I'm black and grew up where nonwhites weren't allowed on public tennis courts. So I had attitude with a capital "A" about this elite sport—I wasn't white and I hadn't worn a size 6 since tenth grade. I was the least likely person to hit the courts.

But my husband bought the racket anyway, along with a gift certificate for lessons with a pro. Despite my reservations, I accepted, asking myself, "How hard can it be to hit a ball over a net? I'll do it, then tell him how boring it is. That will end that."

Guess what? I found tennis to be exciting. It's mental. It's physical. For the first time in my life, I'm part of a team and it's fun, fun, fun! When you meet my teammates later in this book, you'll see why. You'll see how my relationship with each of them has added excitement and self-awareness to my life; how being a part of a team brings people closer together as well as broadens social consciousness. You'll learn how team camaraderie can add spice and purpose to the aging process.

Also, I've developed some "feel good" eating and exercise tricks that I'll share with you, habits I never would have espoused if not for my eagerness to play a good game of tennis. Now, if you're looking for a crash diet and a personal-trainer's routine, expecting to become a Vanessa Williams or Julia Roberts look-alike or to get into that size-eight sweater you wore ten years ago, close this book. That kind of nostalgia will keep you fat and depressed.

Face it, turn fifty and your weight, like your life, will never be the same. Remember the serenity prayer? It goes something like this: "God grant me the strength to accept the things I cannot change, the courage to change the things I can, and the wisdom to know the difference." Heed these words the first time a hot flash wakes you up from a deep sleep and you're sopping wet. And remember them when you notice you've developed a jelly belly that neither sit-ups nor a low-fat diet can budge.

Instead of giving your hips spreading power by settling into the rocker, instead of allowing the second half of your life to drift by on the merits and memories of what you've done, make a change. Don't get stuck in an "oh, Lord, I'm getting old" rut. Change your mental outlook to offset the biological changes. Embrace new challenges. Set new goals. In other words, get a new life. Combine the wisdom gained from your past with a vision to have a blast of a future. This book will show you how the game of tennis and its social outgrowth did just that for me. I hope that my story tickles your funny bone, calms your anxiety about aging, rescues you from the menopause-symptom abyss, and forces you to shift your life's focus from how many years you've lived to how well you intend to live.

PART ONE

Game

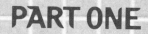

ALICE vs. MENOPAUSE
SCORE: 40/40 (DEUCE)

Who will score the next point?

1

Menopause,
the Reality

I graduated from New Orleans Booker Washington High School in 1966, and my classmates awarded me a black skeleton flag to wave when I was in a bad mood. (Too bad I didn't have that flag when menopause kicked in.) The gift of the flag not only ticked me off, but also hurt my feelings. So I did what the average, you-don't-know-what-you're-talking-about adolecent would do: I declared myself misunderstood. Unfortunately, I transported that defensive perspective into my adult life to call upon whenever things didn't go my way.

Oh, I know. Some Freudian types might suggest that, by ignoring the message my peers offered me, I had built an ego wall to protect my vulnerability and provide the control I craved. Older and wiser, I can't say that I'd disagree with that assessment. But considering my upbringing, self-preservation was tantamount to existing. I was raised by my mother and her mother, who grew up sharecropping on a Louisiana plantation. Plantation women, especially black women, knew their place. They had to be independent as well as dependent, strong as well as tough, nurturing while self-sustaining, intuitive but not introspective.

My mother and grandmother were two such women. They were abandoned by their men in a cosmopolitan city, a short distance yet a long way culturally from their plantation homeland. Thrust into the breadwinner role in a strange work environment, my mama, with her mama's help, struggled to raise two boys and me during that historic period of the 1960s when

women took to the streets, even burned their bras, in their quest
to redefine womanhood.

By the time I was in junior high, I was far more educated
than Mama and Gramma Fun and, as Gramma Fun used to say,
had so much lip it dragged on the ground. I like to say I had
attitude, even though I know now that it worked both for and
against me. Attitude has been the source of my tenacity. With
my take-no-guff personality, I knocked down the doors to get
myself through school, made a career in corporate America, and
survived my first marriage broken by the pain and circumstance
of the Vietnam War. And I lived through years of single parenthood before marrying Frank.

But my attitude was also the source of my fear of failing, of
losing control. And it was attitude that cloaked me in aggression.
With attitude, I was able not only to survive but also to succeed—
to thrive, though outside of myself.

Everyone said I'd inherited Mama and Gramma Fun's independent nature. I thought so, too, until menopause reared its
head. Menopause has a way of forcing you to get in touch with
yourself from the inside out. I found myself asking, am I independent or just afraid? Afraid to really get to know who I was for
fear that others might get to know me, too?

Modeling their own unique version of the Southern belle,
my mother and grandmother taught me how to stay balanced
on life's tightrope, how to be outspoken and secretive, giving yet
selfish, self-reliant while needy. Then menopause set in. And I'm
here to tell you, there's nothing like a couple of years battling
menopausal blues to get a woman off her tightrope and onto the
hard ground. The reality of menopause began its descent upon me
one day like a hailstorm while I stood, of all places, in a grocery-
store checkout line.

I don't know why I decided to go grocery shopping in the
middle of a rainy Saturday afternoon, when the store would be
crowded and the checkout lines were sure to be so long that
they wrapped around one another. The only explanation I have
now is that my mind was in such a state that my procrastination led me straight into desperation. I'd already given procras-

tination art-form status, having gone for days without bread, milk, eggs, coffee creamer, and, Lord help me, toilet paper. With neither paper towels nor tissues in the house, I was out of substitutes.

I forced myself to put down the remote control long enough to get dressed. I'd allowed my household supplies to run out, and now that I think back, it was because I'd abandoned my to-do checklist, a control mechanism that was like a bible to me since the third grade, when I flunked a spelling test.

The day of that test, my teacher, unbeknownst to me, had slipped a note into my lunch bag. It read, "Please teach your child how to spell." Mama and Gramma Fun got hold of the note and I got the whipping of my life. That was the last time I ever misspelled more than one word on a spelling test—and I have the awards to prove it.

But the swatting wasn't the end of my punishment for flunking that test. From that night on, I had to write down every assignment my teacher gave me. Mama, in turn, would check them off the list as I completed them. This kept up through high school. As a result, creating to-do checklists might as well have been innate. So what happened to my reminder to go to the grocery store? As it turned out, my procrastination was symptomatic. But I didn't want to own up to what it was a symptom of.

Back to my grocery-store revelation: There I stood in the checkout line, when I caught a glimpse of my reflection in the glass door of the Coke machine near the magazine rack. I'm five feet, eleven inches tall, and for a pound to show on my broad frame meant that I had to have gained quite a few. Believe you me, the pounds were showing. I had a pooched-out jelly roll for a stomach, and my butt had spread. I couldn't believe how it had spread. Why hadn't I noticed my big ass before? Who had I been looking at in the mirror those past months? Also, I needed a haircut. My chemically relaxed, straight bob had ends that were as frizzy as an Afro—a no-no for me. My mama used to say, "If the hair ain't right, no matter 'bout the rest. You look tacky and ain't fit to go outside." But there I stood, in public, looking like, as Mama used to say, death rolled over.

Remember those television commercials in the fifties, the housewife scrubbing the floor in pearls and high heels? I never went that far, but I certainly was not accustomed to venturing out into public until every hair was in place. What was with me?

I couldn't just stand there in the checkout line looking at this strange version of myself much longer or I'd end up screaming, so I set my sights on the reading material. *Time* and *Newsweek* were sold out, so I picked up a mini book called *Fit and Firm at 40-Plus*. The title of the book didn't set off any bells and whistles in my mind; in fact, I was more likely to wonder about which episode of *Walker, Texas Ranger* I was missing. But then an article entitled "The Menopause Survival Kit: Every Woman's Guide to Perimenopause" grabbed my attention. Why did these words jump out at me? It had to be divine intervention, considering how downright fearful I was of the "M" word.

Are you experiencing any of these symptoms? the article read. *Symptom One: Irregular periods.* Well, I never was regular, I thought. That's why I had my tubes tied at age twenty-eight. *Symptom Two: Heavy menstrual bleeding.* Come to think about it . . . *Symptom Three: Hot flashes.* Hmmm. I'd noticed that, unexpectedly, even when it was cold, my body heated up as if I stepped into a hot sauna. *Symptom Four: Night sweats.* Yeah, I sweat. But that's because Frank has to sleep with those damn blackout curtains drawn in our bedroom. In temperate northern California, that's like closing the windows and turning off an air conditioner, for crying out loud.

I started to put the book down, but I changed my mind. Why? Because I wasn't in a position to be ruling out orders from a higher being here.

Symptom Five: Insomnia. Give me a break, I thought. How can anyone sleep when she's hot? Besides, I'm always too busy thinking about cleaning the garage and rearranging the closets. Who can sleep with ho-hum work like that hanging over them?

I sighed. So far, I'd answered "yes" to all of the symptoms.

"Paper or plastic today?" the cashier asked.

I looked into her dark eyes. Suddenly the urge to cry welled up inside me like an inflating balloon. It was all I could do to keep from bursting right there in the grocery-store line. Me, menopausal? Hell, I wasn't ready to die.

"Are you all right, Miss Alice?" the cashier asked.

"What? Oh. Yes. I'm fine," I said, wishing *Time* and *Newsweek* hadn't been sold out.

The cashier's smile harbored a look of concern. "Paper or plastic this time?" She knew that I alternated between the two.

"Paper."

I read on. *The body- and mind-altering changes caused by menopause* . . . The word "changes" lit me up inside like a bomb wick. I recalled my mama saying that "The Change," as she called menopause, hid horrible diseases in women.

Symptom Six, I read, *Irritability and anxiety or mood swings.* I gritted my teeth. Okay, so I'm uptight. Why wouldn't I be, standing in a grocery line contemplating how long I have to live, wishing I could rip up this book?

Damn.

I turned the page so hard I almost tore it from its binding. Could anger be a menopause symptom, too?

Symptom Seven: Forgetfulness or lack of concentration. Jesus H. Christ. So I forget things. So what? But you forgot to pick Frank up from the airport ten minutes after he'd called to remind you and went to have your nails done instead. I'd thought I was going crazy.

Symptom Eight: Tiredness. Humph. Of course I'm tired. According to this, I'm stressed. I can't sleep. And if my mama was right, I could be dying.

Symptom Nine: Decreased sexual desire. My chest tightened. I tried to remember the last time I didn't just lie there like a bump on a log wishing Frank would finish up. Oh my God, I thought. I'm old *and* impotent.

"Do you want to buy that book?" the cashier asked.

"Buy it?" I whispered.

The moisture of perspiration wet my brow and crawled through the crease between my breasts. Some people giggle when they lie. Well, my sweat glands let loose when I'm agitated.

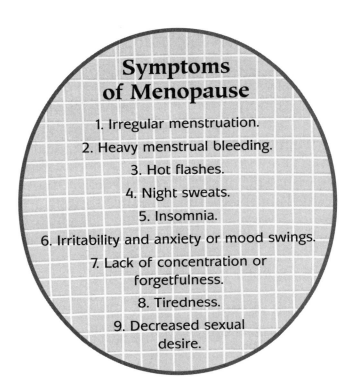

Symptoms of Menopause

1. Irregular menstruation.
2. Heavy menstrual bleeding.
3. Hot flashes.
4. Night sweats.
5. Insomnia.
6. Irritability and anxiety or mood swings.
7. Lack of concentration or forgetfulness.
8. Tiredness.
9. Decreased sexual desire.

"I don't think so."

Why not buy it? my rational side argued. You could use the info.

But I didn't want the info.

I dropped the mini book on the counter, paid my bill, and left. But I carried away with me what I'd read, along with everything else I thought I knew about The Change.

Women makin' the Change got one foot in the grave and one foot out. No tellin' what's really ailin' when a woman makin' the Change.

—MY MAMA

Don't get me wrong, it wasn't as if my mama sat me down and explained menopause. She had a problem talking to me about the facts of life. Why, her explanation of menstruation came in the form of a warning: Keep your legs closed and your drawers up so that some boy won't get to your privates and make you pregnant. But there was always talk—conversations I overheard between her and her friends or statements she made when I had the gall to disagree with her, statements like, "Girl, you sound crazy just like my Auntie Bea when she went through the Change." Her Aunt Bea was a schizophrenic alcoholic. As far as I could tell back then, any change she went through had to do with switching from antagonistic drunk to angelic sober.

I was eight years old, though, when I got the real scoop on The Change. One hot Saturday afternoon, Mama's friend, Miss Zora Mae, wearing that pink chenille robe of hers that was so old the tufted cords running up and down looked like hairy caterpillars, came rushing over from her apartment next to ours. I was sitting between Mama's legs on our front steps getting my recently washed hair braided. I'll never forget how scared I was when I looked up and saw more white than usual in Miss Zora Mae's bulging bug eyes. I started to get up to run, but Mama clamped my body down between her thick knees. I turned my head so that I couldn't see Miss Zora Mae's face, and Mama jerked it back around and whacked me with the comb.

"Juanita," Miss Zora Mae said to Mama, "look at this." She held out a handful of her dyed-red hair.

I'd often heard my mama, a zaftig, five-foot-seven-inch, light-brown-skinned woman, call her very dark friend "Skinny Minnie." When Miss Zora Mae's hand fell from her robe, I could see why. Her ribs were as visible as her garment's protruding pile cords.

"Girl, you must be headed for the Change," Mama said, her tone matter-of-fact.

"The Change? I'm too young for that."

"Girl, hush. This me you talkin' to, not one of them beer-drinking rascals down at Payton's tryin' to get in your pants. You know I know how old you is."

My mama had a flat nose and round cheeks covered with little freckles. I couldn't see her face, pinned down between her legs the way I was, but I could tell by her snippy tone that her freckles were bunched together.

"No need to put my bizness on the street," Miss Zora Mae said, closing her robe, looking around to see if any of the other neighbors sitting on their steps were watching. Gossip was a major pastime in the Magnolia Housing Project.

"All I know is that my Aunt Bea was a little older than you," Mama said. "Fifty-five, I believe, when she started goin' through the Change, and by the time it was over, she was bald-headed. She had to wear a wig to her grave."

My mama's mother, Lucille, my Gramma Fun, died in her mid-fifties, too. My mama would get so lonely for her sometimes, she'd cry. Like the time we were baking jelly cakes for her church's sick and shut-in. Mama was a church stewardess, and on Sundays she and the other women in the group would visit the members who were too ill to attend services.

I liked baking days, not just because of the heated smell of vanilla and pecans that scented our apartment, but because it was always just Mama and me. On baking days I told Mama all about my teachers and school friends, and she told me all about growing up sharecropping in Zachary, Louisiana.

"I wish we woulda knowed," Mama said that day, leaning her hefty frame against the counter, a big crockery bowl hugged under her breasts by one arm.

"Knowed what?" I asked, licking cake batter from my finger.

"Your Gramma Fun thought she was goin' through the Change when what she really had was cancer in her privates. She was just fifty-six years old." Mama wiped her eyes on the tail of her apron. "Women makin' the Change got one foot in the grave and one out. No tellin' what's really ailin' when a woman makin' the Change."

Love/50: Accept what you cannot change.
—MY RATIONAL SIDE

I wasn't as thin as I used to be and the gray hairs were showing, but all in all, I could still pass for thirty-something. Okay, forty-something. But after the grocery-store episode, I felt like an old hag. Perhaps coming face to face with the "M" word two months before my fiftieth birthday triggered an awareness of the old-lady syndrome I'd fallen into. Not only that, everything around me pointed to my getting older. It seemed like incontinence and energy supplements had become the only ads I saw on television and in magazines. More and more of my junk mail promoted senior activities or relief from some old-age ailment. I can't find the words to express the dismay I felt the first time I received an AARP notice addressed to me.

What really knocked me for a loop was a little tête-à-tête I overheard between two women in the beauty salon whose conversations I'd been eavesdropping on for years. For at least a year, I'd listened to them debate whether or not they should get their first blue rinses and exchange their shoulder-length bobs for the shorter, more sophisticated, mature look. For a decade, I'd been entertained by their exchanges, especially on how to bed a man. On this day, however, it wasn't how to bed a man, but how to avoid a man in bed.

"Stay up late sewing or baking or something. You know how quick they fall asleep these days," one woman said.

"You know, what works best for me is an argument. Blame him for doing something stupid and watch him get so mad, he'll volunteer to sleep on the couch."

"Humph. Yeah, you're right. Especially since it doesn't take much to get on the wrong side of me nowadays."

The women chuckled, but I wanted to scream. Could I be closer to their ages than I thought? Am I losing my "womanhood," too? That worry left me feeling naked and stranded on a deserted road. Could I be feeling the same as men who get grumpy and retreat into themselves when they can't get it up?

I panicked. No, I didn't jump up and start pulling out my hair, although I did wonder if it was time for me to get that mature-look haircut the two women had pondered. Instead, the fear burrowed into me on a time-release basis, overwhelming me a little more day by day. I'd conjure up images of myself in a hospital—fat, bald, and dying of cancer.

I needed to slow my whirring mind, but I couldn't. I couldn't pause to consider my circumstance, to deal with the plateau I'd reached in life—I was half of a hundred years old and, in all like-lihood, I wouldn't live fifty years more. I was letting myself be psyched out by the symptoms of an aging female, which were turning me into a first-class wimp and then some.

Take my birthday. Frank and the kids gave me flowers, silk pajamas, and a pair of house slippers. Items, I might add, I took great pains to let them know I wanted.

"I'm turning fifty, not dying," I cried, looking into the beauti-fully wrapped box. "Don't be so hot to stow me away in the bed-room." You would have thought they had given me a burial plot.

My family was flabbergasted by my outburst, by my tears. Hell, I didn't understand me either. How could I expect them to? Especially the tearful me. I'd become a regular waterfall. In all my fifty years, I hadn't cried as much as I did now in a day. Anything and everything could start the flow. And anything and every-thing did. If I turned the key the wrong way and the door would not open, I cried. If Frank spilled water on the kitchen counter, I cried. If I missed an answering-machine message, I cried.

The tears drove Frank crazy. All he could do was retreat—leave the room, the house, the city. Thinking back, I realize that Frank took a lot of get-away trips during that period. And I can see why. "Wimpdom" was so out of character for me.

I've always been a take-charge kind of person. I had to be. My daddy left my mama high and dry with four kids to support. I was the oldest. My mama earned the money, and after Gramma Fun passed on, I took care of our home and my siblings. There was no time to cry and feel sorry. Besides, in the Magnolia Hous-ing Project in New Orleans, there was no crying—just attitude. Attitude when your feelings were hurt. Attitude when you were angry. Attitude when you were sad. Attitude was the only acceptable emotion in the project. Outside of "Attitude Heights," though, I harnessed my emotions by staying in control, being what Frank calls a control freak. Until menopause set in, I had little-to-no experience with the crying affliction.

Why didn't I see a doctor? I should have, I know. I'd seen the commercials, read the magazine articles encouraging women my age to increase their medical visits. I also knew why women didn't heed that advice. Lack of insurance and money head the list. Then there's religion, fear, apathy, lack of enlightenment. None of these affected me. But there I was, fifty years old and I hadn't had my first mammogram. I hadn't had a Pap smear since right after my daughter was born, and she was now twenty. In fact, I didn't step foot in a doctor's office except with my two kids. My distrust was of doctors, not medicine. However, I didn't want my kids deprived of the best health care I could afford, nor did I want to pass my anxiety on to them. The same went for swimming. I am afraid of water, but I made sure they had swimming lessons early on.

It wasn't until menopause had me going when I should have been coming that I told Frank how I felt. Frank, something of a hypochondriac, practically lived in some doctor's office. But he didn't judge me and seemed to understand when I told him that, when I was fifteen, I had a kidney infection that caused me so much pain I ended up in Charity Hospital's emergency room in my native New Orleans.*

"It felt as though someone had taken a hammer to my gut, my stomach hurt so badly," I told him. "I thought I was dying, but the white intern who examined me ordered me not to touch him when I grabbed his arm in agony during the pelvic exam. The way he dismissed my feelings made me feel like the lab rat I was to him."

As a result of that incident, every time I almost talked myself into making a doctor's appointment, I'd think, how can I go through that humiliation again? I'd never make the call.

"With the exception of giving birth," I told Frank, "and the checkups involved during and after pregnancy, I avoid doctors. That experience still haunts me."

"I understand," Frank said.

I don't know why, but I expected more of a lecture from Mr. Healthcare. And when all he said was "I understand" that "what? you don't care?" menopausal paranoia kicked in.

---

*Charity, now University Hospital, remains the training center for Tulane Medical and Louisiana State.

Frank must have sensed from my dazed expression that an argument or perhaps a bout of tears was forthcoming because he picked up a book and his car keys, kissed me, and literally ran from the house.

Thinking back, I guess that Frank, having survived the menopause, illness, and death of his first wife, knew that then wasn't the time to say anything to change my mind about doctors. He knew that desperation would eventually overwhelm me and I'd need assurances, especially from a doctor.

I was reading the newspaper one morning when I saw an article about a substance abuser who had hit bottom, got help, and had just been accepted into a prestigious law school. As I read how she'd lost everything, including the love and support of her family, I thought, could this happen to me? Could I temper tantrum Frank into a divorce? How many sleepless nights can I endure before I lose my mind? How fat do I have to get before I have a heart attack? Am I supposed to end up forever on a couch clutching a television remote?

The alcoholic woman from the article put herself into a substance-abuse program, and according to her, her life began again. She admitted her weakness and moved on. Could I do that? Could I admit that I'd reached middle age and was indeed menopausal? But what did that mean exactly? I knew what it meant to my mama. Thanks to my grocery-store reading, I knew what the symptoms were. However, I didn't have a clue as to whether or not the symptoms could be relieved or how long they lasted. In fact, I really didn't know anything.

I needed information. I needed a doctor, too—maybe even a shrink—but considering my past medical mishap, I had to get the information first. That way I'd have a leg up on what to expect from a doctor.

For me, getting informed has always meant acquiring book knowledge. Since a day long ago in junior high when I had to stay in the library because I couldn't afford a dollar to go on a field trip, the written word has been the fundamental source of my enlightenment. I firmly believe that if not for reading, I might have ended up a benighted hootchie mama in a housing project.

I figured that once I was empowered with book knowledge, I could move on. Then I thought, move on to where? To sixty? To seventy? To the grave? First, move off the couch, I told myself, then head for the library. Reading had steered me onto the right path before. No reason why it shouldn't again.

It was 3:30 P.M. on a school day in early September, and the kids from the nearby middle school filled Rockridge Library like the outside heat. The library building was new, with state-of-the-art computer equipment but few books, and the scent of fresh paint and sawdust was still strong. The double doors sat open to provide air circulation and conserve energy, or so I hoped. Better no air-conditioning than a conservation blackout (common in California during the energy crisis). None of this seemed to bother the kids who rushed in. Their objective, I noticed, was to steal adolescent smooches between the book stacks. For me, however, a blackout would mean that I'd have to breathe recycled paint fumes. But more important, I'd have to use the old-fashioned card catalog. My attention span was way too short these days for that.

I found an empty computer at the research desk not far from the entrance where I could enjoy what little breeze there was, away from the sweaty teens. I entered the dreaded word "menopause." Five hundred and eighty-two listings popped up. Five hundred and eighty-two books written on the deadly subject. Five hundred and eighty-two points of view on the same symptoms. There were clinical books with titles like *Women's Health in Menopause Behavior: Cancer and Cardiovascular Disease* and *Estrogen and Breast Cancer: A Warning to Women*. Could Mama have been right? Was menopause just a disguise or prerequisite for other female diseases?

The spiritual titles included *The Bible Cure for Menopause: Ancient Truths, Natural Remedies and the Latest Findings for Your Health Today; God's Pathway to Healing Menopause;* and *Holy Hormones! Approaching PMS and Menopause God's Way.* Too bad my mama, a born-again Christian, never knew God's take on this female malady. I'm sure she would have touted His remedies as opposed to her own fears and doubts.

For a psychological take, titles ranged from *Change of Life: A Psychological Study of Dreams and the Menopause* to *Mental Disorder and Sexuality in the Climacteric: A Study in Psychiatric Epidemiology.* When I read the book description for the latter title, I decided I'd need a degree in psychology to muddle through this version of the female problem.

The fitness and diet zealots could find words of menopausal wisdom in titles like *Eat Well for a Healthy Menopause: The Low-Fat, High-Nutrition Guide; Eat to Beat Menopause; Outsmarting the MidLife Fat Cell: Winning Weight Control Strategies for Women over 35 to Stay Fit Through Menopause; Menopause and Beyond: A Fitness Plan for Life;* and *Strong Women Stay Young.*

There was even a political publication—*The Menopause at the Millennium: Proceedings of the 9th World Congress on the Menopause.* How's that for governmental perspective?

By the time I'd read the last listing, *Get Off the Menopause Roller Coaster: Natural Solutions for Mood Swings, Hot Flashes, Fatigue, Anxiety, Depression, and Other Symptoms,* I'd sunk deeper into the menopausal abyss.

Finally, I just clicked to get back to the catalog's main menu, looked at the librarian, and said, "Maybe I should just shoot myself and end my misery."

2

The Gift of Life

*Tennis might give you the physical outlet you need to put
some distance between your brain and the hormonal
changes you're experiencing.*

—MY HUSBAND, FRANK

After my experience in the library, I had to concede that I'd
actually reached middle age and was on the threshold of
old age. So how does a person confront such a profound
change? Perhaps I should have chalked up my angst to depression and joined a support group. But I think depression is an
overused word in today's society, an excuse for everything from
a bad-hair day to going on a killing spree. However, since my
mood was persistently disturbed and my relationships were in a
constant state of disruption, I was forced to reckon with the real
culprit—me.

In hindsight, back then I didn't understand where my head
was, where the self-reproach and anger were coming from. I'd
wanted to give up, to get into my rocker and let nature take its
course. That might have worked if I were alone on an island
somewhere. But I wasn't, and the people with whom I came in
contact deserved the courtesy and respect I'd given them before
I became a hormone-lacking, bad-attitude, ranting-and-raving
sister.

I remember having a huge argument with a cable company
representative one day that was so petty I can't recall how it got
started. I do recall, however, telling the young woman that, con-

sidering how incompetent she was, she must've missed at least ten grades of schooling. I said this, mind you, not just to the girl, but to her supervisor as well. How could I have been so callous?

A few days after the confrontation, Frank and I were trying to cool off on the patio outside our living room, Frank relaxing in a chaise, reading, while I checked out the drip-watering equipment servicing the clematis and impatiens around the patio. I relayed my experience with the clerk to Frank and got mad all over again, this time with myself for allowing my insecurity to turn me into the very image of the corporate ogre I'd had to fight in the respect-me battle for years during my career in public relations.

Frank, in that I-hear-you-but-it's-not-interesting-enough-for-me-to-stop-reading way of his, only grunted, while I, on the other hand, scolded myself. Alice, I thought, you've got a serious problem. You didn't have to go off like that. The young woman was pleasant enough, trying hard to do her job. You'd better deal with yourself before you have to get fitted for a straitjacket.

That was only one of many queen-bitch moments menopause put me through. Like the day my daughter, Teasha, and I were driving to the opening of the Great Mall in Milpitas, a town or two away from our home in Oakland. It was a time when Teasha needed patience and understanding more than anything else from me. A simple mother-daughter excursion ended up a car ride in hormone hell.

"Turn right at the next light," Teasha said, closing the guidebook.

I glanced over at my sixteen-year-old. We look alike, Teasha and I, except for skin and eye color. Mine are lighter. Her full rosy lips and pug nose are framed by a perfect oval face covered in smooth, dark chocolate skin—my black diamond.

"That's not what the directions say," I told her.

"I know that, but you didn't turn when you were supposed to. We went too far and had to turn around. Remember?"

"Who do you think you're talking to like that?" I said, unable to ignore the anger bubble that was gurgling in my throat. "You'd better watch how you talk to me before I knock you into king-dom come."

Why was I so angry? The two of us had driven from New Orleans to San Diego when she was twelve, and her map-reading skills were iffy at best. Yet my temperament had been no way near as reactionary as on this fifteen-minute excursion to a new shopping mall.

"I wish you'd try," Teasha mumbled.

I gritted my teeth, pulled the car onto the shoulder of the road, shut off the ignition, and slapped her hard across her face.

Hand in midair, I looked into my daughter's teary, furious eyes and asked myself, what just happened? Better still, why did I do it? Sure, I was upset by Teasha's flippancy but felt more than a little unnerved by the racket from the wheels winding and turning God knows what inside me. And most important, why couldn't I give in to my desire to hug away my child's pain?

If I'd been estrogen sufficient, I would have understood that Teasha and I had experienced a clash of hormones, hers emerg-ing and mine dissipating. And I would've responded like the sane, self-assured parent I prided myself on being.

Menopause initiates awareness of one's own mortality. It gives an aging adult a look inside herself that can be every bit as confusing and frightening as puberty in the adolescent, and even more demoralizing. Especially for someone who has a hard time acknowledging the part of her that's not quite up to stan-dard. After the incident in the car with Teasha, I drove my psyche right into the familiar defensive mode and decided that my new uglies were simply biological, as described in the books I'd read in the library. This is what I told Teasha when I apologized to her a few days later.

The changes in my personality had nothing to do with me per se, I told Teasha. I truly believed that once the biological change was complete, I'd be me again, I'd get back on my tight-rope and take proper care of my family. I didn't see then that, until I confronted the inevitability of nature, I'd exist all right, but as an emotionally challenged individual with a transforming physiology. The biological change I was going through would never be complete if I didn't adapt psychologically.

I'd read or heard someplace that the gift of life is defined by change. Well, change certainly consumed my existence, not to mention my thoughts: change in my body; change in my head; change in my fiery, confrontational attitude; change in the way I treated others—that cable representative, for instance, and my daughter. No wonder my mother was so fearful of The Change. Just hearing the word *change*, no matter the context, sent chills through me. It's strange how a word can have meaning with absolutely no effect until that very word applies to your life's circumstances. Then its meaning strikes you like a bolt of lightning.

Thinking back, I knew something had to give. But I wasn't ready to cross the threshold from young to old, to embrace change and deal with what I thought it meant. Still, I couldn't quash the vision of Gramma Fun pointing her pipe in my face and saying, "Don't get so big for your britches you don't treat people the way you want them to treat you."

So I came up with the usual West Coast mind-body-connect plan to eat more fruits and veggies and to drink plenty of bottled water. For added stress relief, I vowed to take deep breaths before I spoke and to walk my dog, Bonnie, at least four times a week. Not a bad plan, and it did ease my anxiety level. But deep down, I knew I was still a living time bomb.

Frank couldn't help but notice how volatile I'd become. And he understood why, even though I couldn't. A former tennis player, he understood that my life's score was Love/50, and I didn't have a game plan.

Frank was careful about confronting me head-on. He knew better. He'd had prior experience. I'm his second wife, and he's twenty years older than I am. However, in these liberated-woman days, a woman going through The Change can devastate the male psyche more severely than a bra-burning feminist, as I understand his late first wife had been. And there's proven clinical justification for women dumping on men. Remember the 582 books I mentioned? Most were written by men.

Given Frank's previous experience, he suggested that since I wouldn't see a doctor, perhaps I should get involved in some sort of regular exercise, even a sport. And he handed me a tennis racket, a little white pleated skirt, and a gift certificate for two months of lessons with a pro.

Remember the deep breaths? I took several. Inside, I was seething. What the hell was I going to do with a tennis racket? I had issues with tennis.

"You know, Frank," I said in the calmest tone I could muster, "black people and tennis don't go together. I can recall a time when I was a girl, we couldn't set foot on a tennis court. Not even the one in the city public park."

"I'm sure racism was evident back then," Frank said, never looking up from his newspaper. "But that's not what keeps blacks off the court. Not in this day and age."

My mind stalled on the words "back then." I wasn't talking about the Dark Ages. Hell, the Civil Rights Act didn't pass until 1964. It never ceased to amaze me how people seemed to forget that.

"So what does?" I said. "Besides money, that is?"

He'd better not cite the Serena and Venus Williams ghetto-to-tennis-dominance story, I thought. What I'd heard and read about them had convinced me that their success never would've occurred if Richard and Oracene Williams, their parents, hadn't sidestepped the tennis establishment for sponsorship.

"Tennis is considered a sissy sport," he said.

I'd heard that before, too, but I couldn't let him have the last word. "That may be," I said. "But it's an expensive sissy sport. And that keeps not only blacks off the court but other average-wage-earning people, too."

"Let's not argue."

Let's not, I thought. I knew I straddled the thin line between reasonability and that angry-black-woman syndrome that was sure to get me so riled I'd react as if I were still in New Orleans' "Attitude Heights" instead of the Oakland hills.

"Just give the game a try. At the very least, you'll meet women your own age."

I didn't tell him that I believed the only women who played tennis other than the pros and the idle rich were soccer moms with time to kill between carpools.

"Who knows," he said, "it might bring you out of your . . ." His voice trailed off.

He looked at me. Did he see smoke coming from my ears? I could feel the heat on my cheeks. He got up, kissed me on the forehead, and left.

The tennis pro worked from Chabot Canyon Racquet Club, a small place near our house. I'd passed it daily without a thought. I couldn't help but notice the goings-on there now that I had a racket and money tied up in unused training. So I stopped in one day to meet the pro.

I'd never been to a country club before, never wanted to go to a place where people created bylaws to keep out people like me. And even though the racquet club was a small building, a little larger than a two-car garage, I assumed from the name that it was a country club. I walked in expecting to see the tanned, sculpted bodies I'd seen in advertisements and in the movies. Surely, I'd find blond-haired men and women in tennis whites decked out in gold and diamond jewelry, masking their shock at seeing me with a plastic smile.

Instead, I met Katie, a tall, pretty, young woman with long, flowing brown hair, wearing faded gray sweats and an oversized green T-shirt. She greeted me like an old friend. Told me all about the facilities—the six courts, the hot tub out back, the locker rooms and showers, and the diverse ethnic membership of professional men and women. Ordinary people, she said, who play tennis either for fun or competition, but who think it's important to take the time for enjoyment as well as for their health. She explained that Chabot Canyon was neither pricey nor pretentious and that virtually none of the women wore little white pleated skirts. Most members were at least slightly overweight.

Okay, so this was not a little ghetto of the well-to-do. I couldn't throw that in Frank's face. The only thing left was for me to take a crack at hitting a tennis ball over the net. Frank had said tennis was considered a sissy sport. To me, boring was a more accurate description. I'd have to tell him that, but only after I'd given it a try. Why this consideration for him? Because during a rare non-menopausal moment, I decided that I didn't want to hurt his feelings. And when Katie gave me a schedule of the tennis clinics in which I'd been registered and the name and telephone number of the instructor, I felt a twinge of excitement. Could I actually be looking forward to this?

California's rainy season kept me off the courts until early spring, when I had my first tennis experience. It was both humiliating and exhilarating. Remember I told you I'd never played a sport before? Well, that was an understatement. I literally couldn't bounce the ball off the racket, let alone hit it. Every time the ball came my way, I missed it. I touched it a few times. I managed to smash it into the net once or twice. But not once in one and a half hours did I hit that ball over the net—that is, not until my last shot. Then, I wanted to jump up and down shouting and blowing kisses as if I'd just won Wimbledon. But I held back, not wanting to appear foolishly overjoyed at such a small accomplishment.

"You're a natural," one of the women said, patting me on the back, her smile friendly.

A natural disaster, maybe. But, hey, it sure felt good.

"You did better than I did on my first try," she said.

When was that? I thought. When you were a toddler? I knew she was trying to make me feel better, but I couldn't help feeling deprived.

Wendell Pierce, the wiry dark-skinned coach, told me that I'd get better if I kept at it.

I thought about all the times the kids in my neighborhood had taunted me because of my interests: books, movies, and art. How they called me white girl when I didn't even know any white girls to imitate. Will my fellow black menopausal sisters who lived through segregation the way I did think I'm a sellout, too?

"I have no idea what I'm doing here," I told him. "I've never played a sport before in my life. Is it possible to manufacture someone my age into a tennis player?"

He grinned at me and took my racket. "Practice bouncing the ball like this whenever you get the chance," he said, demonstrating how to bounce the ball on the racket strings. "It's a good way to develop hand-eye coordination, to get a feel for hitting the ball in the middle of the racket."

The ball bounced off the racket like the paddle-ball toy that was so popular when I was a kid. I wondered how long it took the other women in the clinic to master that drill—because by the time I could bounce the ball on that paddle three times in a row, my entire adolescence had passed me by.

PART TWO

Set

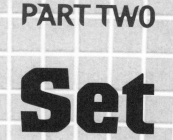

ALICE vs. MENOPAUSE
SCORE: 7/5

I win, but barely.

3

Living on the Mental Edge

Empty wagons make the most noise. You gonna stay in school and fills up your wagon, 'cause a wagon ain't good for nothin' 'less it totin' somethin'.

—GRAMMA FUN

I don't experience all of my life's epiphanies in grocery lines, but supermarket mini-book titles can be so blaring and outrageous, it's hard not to be jolted by them. Here's why I tell you that: After I was blitzed by those titles in the library, and after I began my tennis lessons, I convinced myself that although I still suffered night sweats and mood swings, my life was at last getting back on track. Then one day I had an ice-cream-craving attack. I sold myself on the idea that the orange sherbet/lite vanilla ice cream swirl I had in mind was low-fat enough that it wouldn't add too many more pounds to my ever-expanding behind. And I went to Albertson's supermarket. There I wound up at the tail end of what seemed like a half-block-long express line, reading the following in Ronald Klatz and Robert Goldman's mini book *Fight Aging:* "Mental fitness declines with age. Dementia, memory loss and the inability to concentrate are some of the results."

I swear I suffered a mild heart attack when those words flashed before my eyes—words that became absolutely, without a doubt, the scariest aspect of getting older that I'd processed so far. I hurriedly put the book back on the shelf, as if replacing it would relieve the tightness I felt in my chest.

Dementia . . . The word played over and over in my head like a broken record, getting me so flustered I could hardly breathe. But like a battered woman who is as much afraid to leave as she is to stay, I picked up the book and read on.

Supermarket mini-book information is limited. That's why they're called "mini books," I guess. But they do whet the appetite for more facts. For instance, *Fight Aging* cited a study that found that mental acuity stays high if the brain is continually challenged. Okay, I thought after I read this, what exactly does "continually challenged" mean? Playing Scrabble? Doing crossword puzzles? These sounded like old-folks-home activities to me. Needless to say, that morsel of information was about as gratifying as Diet Coke is thirst-quenching. The carbonated beverage works until you take the last swallow. Then there's the lingering aftertaste that only another drink will dissipate. By no means did this mini-book tidbit remove the afterthought the word *dementia* had imprinted on my brain.

So I headed back to the library to further examine a few of those 582 books on menopause. Some author must have realized that some 20-million-plus women would soon be entering menopause; some 20-million-plus women forgetting the name of the offspring they're addressing, forgetting their house and telephone numbers. Publishers must know that the baby-boomer stampede is underway, and for the next twenty years or so, those of us in our fifties and sixties will need information on how to live on the mental edge.

The library was calm. As I looked around, it dawned on me that the Saturday 10 A.M. hour must be the old-timers' slot, as opposed to the Friday 3 P.M. after-school puberty hour. Two wrinkled and stooped women leaning on walking canes stood in the checkout line sharing whispers over a terribly worn copy of Jane Austen's *Pride and Prejudice*, a favorite of mine since junior high. The weak-kneed moment I experienced flitted by but was nonetheless disconcerting. Could this be me? When? Next year? The year after, maybe?

The fluorescent daylight flowed in like a cascading waterfall through the wall-to-wall, ceiling-to-floor windows and shone on the two women like a stage light. I squeezed my eyelids closed, hoping to vanquish the elderly women into darkness along with the vision of myself, decrepit and engaged in conversation with them. Slowly I opened my eyes but looked away, afraid that I might experience another senior Kodak moment.

Lord, I'm way too young to relate to these people. I quickened my step, heading toward the card-catalog computer.

When I reached the computer, I typed in the keyword "menopause" and took a deep breath. A lot of questions about menopause rolled around in my head. Some answers I wanted and some I didn't. I was sure I didn't want to confirm my mama's take on estrogen loss. That would mean I was knocking on death's door. Lord knows I wasn't prepared to go there.

I decided to focus my hunt for information on the memory-loss aspect, hopeful that the research done on that facet of menopause would provide not just fleeting, flimsy ideas, but studies that proved that forgetfulness and memory loss were two different things, a distinction that had to be made clear to me, because how many times in a day did I misplace not just my car keys but, say, a glass I'd been drinking from before going into the bathroom? The newspaper I picked up to read before answering the phone? My eyeglasses? I desperately wanted that paragraph I'd read on memory loss in *Fight Aging* to be as insubstantial as the tabloid headlines on the rack next to it.

Finally, when the massive oak library table was covered with books devoted to menopause, as many as I could locate on my three trips to the shelves (and almost as many as the new library had), I flipped through the contents pages. Every title had an entire chapter on memory loss.

With a butterfly running amok in my stomach, I proceeded to educate myself. The first sentence I read said that memory malfunction doesn't usually occur until the very late stages of the aging process.

"That'll work," I said aloud, "if my late stage is somewhere between ninety-five and a hundred."

I talked to myself all the time. The voice in my head I spoke to started off as the invisible friend I'd conjured up to keep me company when I was a child. It grew up with me, continuing to be my sounding board when I was alone or too unsure of myself to share what was on my mind with a real person.

"I should be ready to shut down by a hundred."

"Shhhh."

I followed the sound across the room to the spectacled, reedy, dirty-blond librarian standing behind the research desk. Our eyes met, and I saw her put her index finger across her lips the way my mean-spirited third-grade teacher, Miss Trout, used to do. I resisted the childish temptation to give her the finger, remembering how encouraging my junior-high-school librarian had been. I smiled at her instead.

"I lay odds she's a boomer," I whispered, lowering my head into a book. "Lord knows I understand what that's done to her disposition."

I picked up another book and read that some scientists and doctors believe that much of what can go wrong with your mind and body as you age is hereditary.

"Jesus." My voice rose with excitement.

I glanced over at the librarian. She frowned. I frowned right back at her, thinking, what's her problem? There was no one around to disturb.

That hereditary stuff was alarming. My maternal and paternal grandmothers all died from some form of cancer. And Papa, my great-grandfather, who lived to be ninety-eight, give or take a few years, was as nutty as a fruitcake. When he wasn't pinching the butts of young girls (including me), he was strutting around with a Civil War musket to guard his money and his home from the Klan. And there was my second cousin Nonie, and my nephew—both wonderful, both born mentally challenged.

Estrogen deficiency, I read on, can also be the cause of mental dysfunction. For fifty years I've lived with estrogen and hadn't heard it or seen it written enough to learn to spell it. Now, because it's diminishing, I find out that not only could I be dying, but I could possibly lose my mind?

Consider the time a few months earlier when I went to the DMV to renew my driver's license. I started to fill out the form and couldn't recall the year I was born. I don't mean it just slipped my mind, either. For the life of me, I couldn't remember it. I tore up the half-filled-out document and fled. My emotions ran, too—from "Oh, my God, what the hell is the matter with me?" to anger at myself for being a ninny about common human forgetfulness.

Sometimes I'd have to read a paragraph, I don't know how many times, before I understood it. I'd go into the pantry to get a can of soup or something and find myself staring around trying to figure out why I was there. I wondered, are there loony wards in old-folks homes?

From my research, I learned that estrogen receptors exist throughout the brain to direct brain-cell signals for functions such as emotions, moods, thinking, body heat, and sex drive. All that? If the estrogen in my body is on the decline, I worried, so is my life. But then I read in *The Wisdom of Menopause*, by Dr. Christiane Northrup, that further confirmation is needed to determine the correlation between estrogen and brain function; she noted that memory problems at midlife can be due to temporary overload from many external demands on—get this—"limited time."

Well, isn't a menopausal woman's time limited? Of course the brain is overloaded with thinking. No wonder I was fuzzy-headed.

"The brain doesn't have to degenerate," another author wrote. "Its design feature is such that it should continue for a lifetime."

Oh, yeah? I thought. Then what's with the memory loss? With dementia? With Alzheimer's?

What can I say? The lack of estrogen and the lapsed-memory connection tormented me. I worried about having way too many "senior moments," as these memory lapses have been dubbed, and I practically OD'd on stress when I added thoughts about my demented great-grandfather. Talk about vulnerable.

When I was estrogen sufficient, I would rather sleep on a bed of nails than succumb to these kinds of feelings. But how could I be confident about anything, afraid as I was that I could lose my mind at any minute? After all, thanks to Gramma Fun, the development of my mind was the source of my self-confidence.

I'll never forget my first major lesson on the power of self-belief. After we'd moved from a two-room flat on Dupre Street to the luxurious Magnolia Housing Project, indoor plumbing and all, I had to go to a new school. On the first day, I encountered the school bully, a tall, overweight, dark-skinned girl named Lena Bell Wilcox. Lena Bell came up to me at lunchtime and ordered me to give her my three cents for milk and half of my sandwich. First of all, I drank water with my lunch so that I could save my pennies. I wanted to buy a pair of shoes so that I would no longer have to wear my mama's shoes stuffed with paper to fit. Second, I had a mayonnaise-and-sugar sandwich. No way was I going to let her and the other kids know that we couldn't afford sandwich meat. So when Lena Bell followed me into the girls lavatory to continue to intimidate me, I flushed her head in the toilet. Her braids got caught in the commode, and the janitor had to cut them to pull her head out.

The vice principal gave me detention and would have suspended me if my fellow classmates hadn't told story after story about how Lena Bell had been bamboozling them since kindergarten. Her reign of schoolyard terror ended that day, but not before she told everyone that I had to eat mayonnaise-and-sugar sandwiches for lunch.

I went home determined never to show up at Thomy Lafon School, or any other school, ever again. When I told all of this to Gramma Fun, she got ready to tell me the empty-wagon story.

She drew her George Washington tobacco from her white vinyl purse and removed its blue foil wrapper, getting ready to smoke her pipe. Smoking and storytelling generally went together, unless Gramma Fun also pulled out her Bible. That meant she wanted her quiet time with the Lord.

I followed my grandmother into the kitchen, a room barely big enough for the double sink and the hot-water heater that sat between the apartment-sized stove and the small refrigerator. I sat across from her at the bright yellow Formica table that was flush against the army-green, grease-stained wall. Gramma Fun removed her pipe from her apron pocket, stuffed it with tobacco, and lit up. I watched her puff the smoke in and out, her lips popping with each exhale. I was determined to give her every courtesy, including a forced laugh. Usually, even Gramma Fun's sad stories made me laugh. That's why I called her Gramma Fun. But the day's events had left me feeling so low that I didn't believe that any of her fables, no matter how witty, would be able to cheer me up.

She pulled the pipe from her lips and waved it at me.

"Now you listen to me," she said, her tone no-nonsense. "When I was a li'l girl, every Sunday, me and my mama and my brothers and my sisters, all of us would help Papa load up his wagon with all the 'tatoes and corn and greens and sugar cane from the field it could carry. Then Papa went to town to sell it. When Papa pulled that full wagon down the road, we ain't heard nothing. But when night fall, and it was time for Papa to come home, we sat quiet as mouses, prayin' to hear that ole' wagon chugglin' up the road."

Gramma Fun took a long draw from her pipe, her dark brown eyes fixed on me, mine on her.

"Papa used to all the time say 'empty wagons make the most noise.' Now, you see them chaps who teasin' you?" she said. "Them chaps got empty wagons. You gonna stay in school and you gonna fills up your wagon, 'cause a wagon ain't good for nothin' unless it totin' somethin'."

In the library, remembering Gramma Fun's pep talk made me feel that if my mind went, I'd be like an inmate on death row, a dead woman walking.

"Gramma Fun," I sighed, "I hate to tell you this, but a mind ain't good for nothin' if it can't remember what it's totin'."

If the librarian had appeared right then to chastise me for

conversing with Gramma Fun, we would have had words. I was way past self-control. Personal reflection, I realized, didn't always produce strong, positive psychological results.

Why does nature forsake women this way? I wondered. And in today's high-tech world, it's easy to replace body parts—knees, shoulders, hips, even eyes. But brain replacement? Perhaps Gramma Fun's assessment of female physical maladies from menstruation to childbirth is the only answer: that female nature is the punishment cast upon women because Eve gave Adam that damn apple to eat.

I stared down at the books, thinking that the mess on the table was as telling as the mess going on inside of me. The books were supposed to straighten out my thoughts, but I couldn't relate to what I'd read. The information painted a self-portrait as intimidating to me as high-school calculus problems had been and no clearer. I couldn't find those answers, and I couldn't find me. The only thing I knew for sure was that the person I'd become feared living as much as she feared dying.

I propped my elbows on the table and held my head between my hands.

"That's what you get for being inspired in a supermarket," I said, aware of the echo of my voice.

I looked around for the librarian. She wasn't there. I was alone with the estrogen-deficient mass of confusion that had taken over my body. I knew that if I wanted to see myself in the mirror again, I'd have to accept the fact that I'd lived long enough to make The Change. What that meant exactly I still hadn't figured out. I took a deep breath. My only certainty was that I had to keep my soul alive, to rescue my womanhood. How? Now that was another matter.

My brain took in a lot of facts about menopause. But the facts didn't scale the walls of denial and fear that surrounded me. I remained overwhelmed by the prospect of a demented future. When I got home, I did what I'd heard most people do these days when they want more than facts, when they need insight to help seal their grip on something. I clicked on to the

Internet, a chat room no less—another indication that time had caught up with me.

A while back I'd read an article about how the Internet was fast becoming a companion, a connection to the present, for older people. I surmised, therefore, that chat-room communication was a lifeline for lonely, elderly people too afraid to connect physically with the world outside the sanctity of their homes or, heaven forbid, their institutions. I know now this was an irrational reaction, but when menopause became a reality, anything relating to the aged, no matter how insignificant, took on monumental implications.

I ended up asking strangers I could neither see nor hear if they knew of something medical, some pill or herb I could take, that would keep my mind intact. A woman who called herself Odessa told me that estrogen replacement therapy (also known as hormone replacement therapy, or HRT) had shown good results in increasing short-term memory and enhancing the ability to learn new tasks.

I'd read this, of course, but for some reason, those written words didn't play their usual magic on me. I'd even seen a popular actress's commercial advocating HRT many times on television. Boy, was I deep in denial. I thanked God that Odessa made HRT clearer to me, and decided to seek out that treatment. But then another woman warned me that the estrogen pill could increase my cancer risk.

"Jeez," I cried out, "can I get a break here?" I'd spent forty of my fifty years in environmentally unsafe Louisiana breathing Good Hope Refinery air. Throw in the hereditary factor, and I was already a cancer risk.

"You know, Alice . . . ," the woman wrote. For some reason, seeing my name on the computer screen like that, I felt silly and exposed. I thought, I probably shouldn't have given my real name.

I read on, "You must know that stress is a lifestyle factor that contributes to many adverse menopausal changes, including zapping memory power. If you don't want to give yourself a coronary or end up in an early grave or some mental institution, chill out and carefully explore your options."

My fingers flew across the keyboard. "Who are you, lady," I wrote, "some voodoo stress detector?"

If ever there was a time for me to take a deep breath, that was it. I pressed down on the delete key and typed in the word "thanks," wondering how a woman I communicated with via cable could possibly sense how stressed out I was.

I got off the computer thinking, if only I could talk to Gramma Fun. But she died before she had time to process her own menopause experience. And an accident followed by a leg amputation and a tainted blood transfusion had claimed Mama before she was old enough to feel comfortable discussing the subject with me.

I had an urge to bawl like a hungry baby and sought refuge in the garage/laundry room. Not because it was such a great place—it wasn't, all dust and cement, stuffed with junk and the dirty clothes I'd brought down a few days earlier—but because it was out of Frank's earshot. I plopped down on top of a Sears toolbox and let go—hacking, racking crying that made my face ugly with a runny nose, drooling mouth, and red eyes.

I don't know how long I sat alone in the garage, trying to divert my thinking from the apprehension that engulfed me. I told myself that I had a knack for blowing things out of proportion, especially with my hormones on a runaway train. I even tried to redirect my concentration (a trick I'd learned in Psych 101) to the spider building a web in the narrow space between the washer and dryer. But when I thought about how often I'd swept that web away, I felt jealous of how determined and in control that spider was.

The next morning, around 2:30 A.M., I woke from a restless, dream-filled sleep looking as if I'd been in a wet T-shirt contest. The crazy dreams affected me more than the night sweats—not because I remembered any specific dream details, but because I sensed they were gory. My anxiety made me fear closing my eyes despite my need to get a good night's sleep.

I'd scheduled a tennis lesson for 7:30 that morning. At any time later, mental as well as emotional exhaustion would have

turned me into a zombie. This was particularly disturbing because over the weeks I'd grown to enjoy tennis in spite of my
advanced age and lack of sports savvy and background. I can't
explain how that happened. I'd read about exercise junkies and
the zone they strived to get into. I don't know if that's what I
experienced or not. I only know that when I was on the court, I
wanted to be as sharp as possible. I had to work really hard to
remember basic instructions like "turn your shoulders and split-
step on the ball-bounce." Tennis worked my nerves from one
lesson to the next. I needed to be rested. I didn't want the tennis
ball to get the better of me.

"Go to sleep," I said, rolling over. I pushed the covers aside
and hugged a pillow. I closed my eyes and tried to envision myself moving like Venus on the court. Sports therapists call this
learning tactic "visualization." But all I could visualize was Coach
Wendell hitting balls to me and me returning them right into the
net. I punched the pillow, resituated my head, and dozed off again.

"Keep your feet moving and go to the ball." I could hear Coach
Wendell's instructions in my subconscious. He hit me another
ball. I lifted one foot, then the other. I dumped the return into
the net. I hadn't moved forward, only stepped in place. My brain
had told my feet where to go, but they wouldn't budge. Even in
a dream, there's no worse feeling than knowing you're doing the
wrong thing while you're doing it and are helpless to do what
you know is right.

I turned again, careful not to disturb Frank, snoring loudly
beside me. "Sleep," I whispered. "Tired minds cannot outthink or
outrun tennis balls."

Once again, I closed my eyes and drifted off. But seeing
myself swirling around in a wheelchair in a dark hole without
eyeballs was the last straw. That wasn't sleep, nor was it dream-
ing. It was agony, so I got up.

Besides, I rationalized, old-lady tennis players don't run
down balls; they slice and dice them off the racket with so much
spin, Wilma Rudolph couldn't get to them.

"Mindless TV. That's what I need," I said, snuggling under a
blanket in my easy chair. I tuned the television to the Love chan-

nel to watch *The Thornbirds* for the umpteenth time. "Nothing frightening about a priest having an affair, right?"

I glanced at the coffee table and spotted a book I'd checked out of the library, *Successful Aging* by Drs. John W. Rowe and Robert L. Kahn, about the MacArthur Foundation Study on aging in America. I had browsed through it earlier and recalled seeing something about physical fitness being strongly linked to cerebral fitness in the aged. The concept barely touched a chord in me at the time, but thinking about my tennis lesson and the state of my mental health brought it back to mind.

According to the study, older people who are physically active have good lung function and are likely to maintain sharp mental ability because the brain is getting the oxygen it needs to be healthy.

"Think of the brain as a muscle that needs exercise to stay fit like all muscles," I read out loud. "Mental acuity stays high if the brain gets exercise."

Brain fitness? Sounds like an infomercial.

"A mental exercise," I read, "is anything that makes one think. A memory tool is something that controls and organizes information to be remembered. Such organization lessens forgetting and can be fun."

For the first time since the word "menopause" had invaded my psyche, I paused. Why, a tennis player has to remember a dozen steps just to hit the ball: Get in ready position. Adjust the grip. Follow the ball. Split-step on the bounce. Keep the feet moving. Bend the knees. Move to the ball. Turn the shoulders. Keep your eyes on the ball until it hits your racket. Remember your sweet spot. Pick a target. Follow through on your shot.

Talk about boosting brainpower.

Mama used to tell me all the time that there is no power like mind power. "If people call you stupid and you believe 'em," she'd say, "you stupid. But if you think you're smart, no matter what people say, you smart."

I'd granted menopause power over my mind, which in turn controlled my personal constitution and zapped my energy. No wonder I felt old and hopeless.

I looked heavenward. "When you think you're old, you're old. Mind power, huh, Mama?"

What Mama called mind power is called "mental toughness" in tennis. I'd heard the term before, but it really clicked in my head when I recalled my mama's words. Funny how something old can help you relate to something new. I felt as though a veil had been lifted from my eyes. I smiled at the good feeling that surged through me. Could tennis become my ticket to mental longevity?

According to Scott Perlstein, author of *Essential Tennis*, the mental aspects of the game of tennis are effort, focus, and discipline. Or, in the words of my mama, "If you don't want nothin', you won't get nothin'."

Perlstein wrote that what really makes a tennis player a winner is attitude. He said that a good tennis player walks onto the court believing she will win. Mama said that when you look in the mirror, you better like what you see; for those who don't, remember it's their problem, not yours. Attitude? Damn straight.

If only I could apologize to Venus Williams for agreeing with her critics when they called her cocky after she'd whipped Martina Hingis in the 2000 U.S. Open semifinal. During that match, Venus fought off attack after attack, strategy after strategy, and won because, in her own words, "I knew that I could."

Tennis, I began to understand, could very well help me develop that same kind of mental stamina, exactly what I needed to overcome the menopausal attack on my confidence. I'd noticed that even with my limited exposure to the game so far—lessons with Coach Wendell and hitting against the backboard—while I was playing tennis, I forgot all the stuff that slowed me down off the court. I forgot my age, how fat I was, how wimpy. The only thing that mattered was whether or not I could hit the ball with more purpose than I did the last time I tried. It stood to reason that if I could improve my performance on the tennis court, those gains could well translate into a far better, more confident life off the court. This notion became my reality when I read in *Successful Aging* about memory experiments that showed that once older people are convinced of their ability, they devote more time and effort to memory tasks as well as to physical fitness, and thus attain further gains in both performance and self-esteem.

As serendipity would have it, once I recalled Mama's philosophy of self-awareness, I began to shed the menopause cloak of denial. I became more receptive to the information the books were feeding me about aging in women.

For instance, unless there is some sort of brain illness, like an inoperable tumor, a person rarely forgets how to turn on the television or drive a car. These activities are guided by what is called "working memory," or the learned routine on which we rely in our daily lives. Working memory shows little, if any, decline with age. It's more likely that an older person will lose her physical ability to perform routine tasks rather than forget how.

The memory we may or may not lose during menopause is called "explicit memory"—the intention and the ability to instantly recall a telephone number or a birth date. This is not the kind of memory loss that puts you into a rocker or gets you locked up.

Whew! Believe me, knowledge is spelled R-E-L-I-E-F. The thought of living without mental control after depending on it so heavily all my life had me thinking about when would be too soon to contact an assisted-death doctor.

And the Doctor
Said . . .

The truth is, the more we sit on our buns stressing over
getting old, the fatter, sicker, and older we make ourselves.

—MY DOCTOR

Weeks passed. I learned to hit the ball over the net with some regularity. But the thrill of this accomplishment didn't stop me from feeling as if I were riding around with an expired license plate. New physical ailments emerged, compounding my menopausal vulnerability. Along with a lingering feeling that I was sinking in quicksand, my entire body hurt.

I'd expected the muscle aches and pains. After all, I had never been this physically active before. But the chest pains, the constipation, and the fatigue kept me throbbing while in a perpetual state of panic. Could Mama have been right? Could there be some disease lurking around inside of me pretending to be menopause?

Concerned as I was about such possible illness, I stuck with tennis. I was hooked. Go figure. I attended professional matches, watched them on television, learned the names of players, selected favorites. I even learned to keep score. All of this made me feel even more like a used-up dishrag the day I got yet another in-your-face, you're-an-old-lady reminder. This time it was my teeth with a condition requiring my dentist to refer me to a periodontist.

What does visiting a periodontist have to do with my consti-

pation and fatigue? Nothing, really, but one has to start these
little vignettes from the beginning or they lose their oomph in
the telling.

Anyway, as I recall, the day was wet, and the cold weather
mirrored my gloomy spirit. I couldn't stop thinking that not
only was I getting old, but I might also have gum disease. Talk
about rocker-ready. I envisioned my toothless, flabby, fat body
sitting on the porch of some old-folks home, gumming down
strawberry Jell-O.

A steady rain pounded my car's window and blurred my
nearsighted vision as I drove around looking for the periodontist's office. The signage—I noticed after I'd parked and run into
the two-story building I thought I was looking for—didn't match
the address numbers I'd been given. I ended up in a clinic for
women. Divine intervention? What, again?

I looked around for someone to direct me to where I had to
go. The space was small but neat. The walls and furniture were
in shades of white, mauve, and green, oozing femininity and
warmth as well as strength. I noticed the freestanding bookshelf
and the magazine rack right away. It was not the usual waiting-
area coffee table strewn with copies of last year's *Reader's Digest*
and *People* magazines.

"I'll be right with you," the receptionist said before disap-
pearing into a back room.

I nodded, thinking the wait would give me a chance to dry
off and peruse the bookshelf. I love checking out the books on
other people's shelves. I pride myself on being able to tell a lot
about people by what they read. Take religious books, for example. If someone's shelves are full of books on various religions,
then according to my deductions, the reader is a student or an
intellectual. Or an atheist trying to disprove the Immaculate
Conception theory. The religious reader, I believe, would simply
keep those books specific to her faith: copies of the Bible, the
Koran, or the Torah, and titles on how to read and understand it.

The reader who has only mysteries and thrillers may be
bored or dissatisfied with her life's status quo and likes the

escapades and adventures of characters who tread in and out dangerous situations.

But the reader who reads everything is on a mission. She wants to be able to say that she's read "x" number of books and to be able to reference her reading on any given topic. She will probably like stories written by Danielle Steel but will boast about having enjoyed the genius of Tolstoy. I read everything.

On the shelves in this office, however, were books on breast cancer, heart disease, childbirth, and women's sexuality; exercise books; books on nutrition; books on Western and Eastern clinical treatments for female problems, including—you guessed it—menopause. There were newsletters and periodicals on women's health that I'd never seen before.

"Sorry about that," the receptionist said. "How can I help you?"

"What is this place?" It wasn't your everyday doctor's office, that's for sure. And the mystery of why and how I'd gotten there continued to prey on my thoughts.

"This place?" The woman did a quick sweep of the space with a glance around, a where-do-I-start look on her face. I did a quick sweep over her casual outfit: jeans and a cream-colored cotton T-shirt. Her skin was clear, seemingly makeup-free, though her cheeks were rosy and her lips red. She reminded me of the girl in the Pond's cold cream ads back in the sixties.

Finally she said, "A group of women doctors got together and started this practice to place emphasis on women's health issues, and . . ."

"Women doctors?"

Of course I knew there was such a mammal. But coming from the South and having been raised in the true Southern tradition, where women were taught that men had all the answers, it never occurred to me to seek a woman doctor for what ailed me.

"All of our doctors and aides are female. Would you like an appointment?"

I hesitated. It's strange how traditions, even those with which we disagree, get molded into our way of life.

The receptionist must have thought I was crazy, the way I just stood there, staring at her as if she were a being from another planet. If she only knew that at that moment I was kicking myself for not having read *Men Are from Mars, Women Are from Venus*.

"Here," she said. "Take this. Read it through." She handed me a little packet of papers. "If you're interested, fill out the medical information and call me. My name is Trudy. I'll get you an appointment right away."

"Okay, I will," I said and walked toward the door. I didn't even bother to ask her about the periodontist's office. Instead I stared at the paperwork she'd given me, making sure that my wishy-washy memory recorded this meeting for future reference.

I went out to the street and, like magic, saw the marquee that directed me to the periodontist offices on the floor above. I was in the right place after all.

The periodontist turned out to be a really cute Asian-African American with a quarterback body and a Marcus Welby manner. He told me that although I had gum problems, they were by no means so bad that I'd have to have my teeth extracted.

"How did this happen?" I asked. "I brush and floss daily."

"How old are you?"

"What does that have to do with my teeth?" my voice rose. Was every part of my body going to fall apart just because I'd turned fifty?

The young man looked up at me. I could see that he didn't quite know how to respond to my reaction.

"Nothing," he said, "except preventive dental care and services were not always available to . . . to . . ." He averted his gaze.

"To blacks? You can say it," I told him. "And, yes, I'm old enough to remember that. When I was growing up in New Orleans, a white dentist, whose office was on First and Claiborne, was the only dentist willing to work in our part of town."

The young man's astonished expression spurred something in me. For some reason, I was upset that he knew about the time when blacks didn't get adequate dental care but was ignorant as to why.

"Would you believe that I didn't know a black dentist until I moved to California?"

The young man opened his mouth to speak, but I didn't wait.

"When I was a little girl," I said, "on Saturdays I used to go window shopping at the TG&Y on Claiborne Avenue. I saw people lined up down the block, holding their swollen faces and waiting for that white dentist to pull out their pain, the only dental service he provided. He charged a quarter a tooth."

The young man's shoulders dropped, and he turned away to his computer.

"Yes, ma'am," he whispered.

I felt bad for putting him through that, more so for dredging up that memory. My brother was practically toothless because of that tooth-pulling practice. And I'd suffered many a toothache so as not to end up that way.

"Ma'am, since it takes years for teeth and gums to go bad," the young periodontist said, "it's gonna take years to get them healthy."

"Years, huh?" Well, suppose I don't have years? I couldn't argue this with the young man, so I smiled.

When I left the periodontist's office, I carried with me a Soni-Care electric toothbrush, a Waterpik, a series of brushes and picks to clean my gums, a stannous fluoride rinse, and six months of deep-cleaning appointments. The periodontist told me that this aggressive treatment would keep me from having my teeth extracted, and I could possibly avoid gum surgery. That's when I decided to make an appointment at the women's clinic. If I was headed over the hill, I was going on my terms—with my own hair and my own teeth.

Two days later I greeted the female doctor. She was in her early fifties, a sixties throwback with long, graying reddish brown hair, a flowing flowered skirt, and, oh yeah, Birkenstocks. What I call an official hippie.

We shook hands and I felt something. Call it an electric current, a jolting sensation. I don't know how to describe it without sounding like a poet hung up on adjectives. But I definitely felt a vibration in spite of my defensive and cool demeanor. I'd put my aggressive "projects" attitude in check, ready to expose it only if the lady doc turned out to be a female version of her insensitive male peers.

I wanted to know right off if I could let my guard down, so I rushed to tell her about my humiliating teenage experience with a physician, and how that experience had festered and poisoned my opinion of doctors over the years.

"That's why my two colleagues and I started this clinic," she said, leaning back in the chair, her attention focused on me. Me, not my medical questionnaire and not her notepad. She shared herself with me as if I were interviewing her, as if what I thought would make a difference to her.

"We found that too many women felt uncomfortable exposing themselves to men, or felt that their male physicians didn't really understand their ailments," Doc said. "Worse, that they didn't care to understand them."

"No," I said. "The worst, in my opinion, is when you leave with a nod, a fake smile, and no help." I'd heard from lots of women who had experienced that degradation.

Doc nodded. "Yes. As a result, women either don't go for regular checkups or don't disclose fully any discomforts they're experiencing."

I sighed. This woman with the flower-child compassion and prep-school intellect had put me at ease.

"That's particularly true with women our age." Doc's eyes were still glued to mine.

"Menopausal women," I whispered, as though I'd released an uncomfortable gas bubble.

"That's correct."

Her smile said it all. She understood, so the "gab" exam began. We talked for over an hour. The lady doc took the time to answer all of my questions with the wisdom of a person who'd been there and the attention of a skilled, professional caregiver who gave a damn. I never imagined I could have such interaction, such dialogue, with a medical person.

I felt so comfortable talking with Doc that I gave her an account of my family's medical history that far exceeded the traditional medical questionnaire. I told her all about my great-aunt Bea, about my grandmothers, and about how my mother believed that menopause symptoms hid the diseases that would kill them until it was too late.

Doc explained that the seeds for cardiovascular disease and diabetes could be sown when levels of estrogen decrease, that estrogen-deficient women are more susceptible to obesity, high blood pressure, and high cholesterol. All of these can trigger cardiovascular and other serious diseases.

"So my mama was right?"

"Well, let's say it's true that women do tend to develop heart disease later in life. But there is much that can be done to prevent that from happening."

"Diet and exercise," I mumbled.

"You say that like they're bad words. The truth is, the more we sit on our buns stressing over getting old, the fatter, sicker, and older we make ourselves. Especially if we compound a non-active lifestyle with cigarette smoking, alcohol, and overeating."

"My great-aunt Bea smoked several packs of Winstons a day. My dad's mom had diabetes and weighed close to three hundred pounds."

"Stands to reason then that your grandmother and your aunt rushed their deaths along."

"But my other grandma, she wasn't fat and she . . ." My voice trailed off. "She had uterine cancer. And my mama . . ."

"I'm sorry," Doc said. She looked me dead in the eyes and patted my hand. I still felt like crying, but I smiled instead, grateful not to have to go into details while I fought off tears.

Doc had me undress then and ushered me up onto the table for my physical. I was so relaxed I hardly felt the "duck bill" inserted for the pelvic exam. And the breast exam was a combination checkup and training on proper technique for self-examination. What a relief it was not to feel like some man was feeling me up under the guise of looking for lumps.

"What about cancer?" I asked. "My mama was scared to death

of going through the Change for fear she'd get uterine cancer like her mama."

"Cancer risks are not higher during the transitional years."

"They're not? But I thought . . ."

"You thought that when your body ages, your internal defenses are weakened, or some old wives' tale like that."

"Yeah, something like that."

"It's true that in cancer, cells change. But that's because genes control all aspects of cell life. And as time passes and we age, genes may change. But that change can be brought on by breathing bad air or cigarette smoke, from exposure to environmental carcinogens like pesticides, from consumption of alcohol, preservatives, and even fatty foods."

"Or God's will." My mama's dying words.

"I'm not qualified to consult on God's intentions."

I left the women's clinic having opted to undergo HRT. Armed with a prescription for the wonder hormone, estrogen, and a newfound respect for doctors, I had high hopes that I would soon have my sanity back. But my symptoms persisted. The anxiety, irritable mood swings, and insomnia remained. Not to mention the weight gain, despite my increased physical activity. What scared me as well as ticked me off was my chronically dry and brittle hair and nails. My mama had instilled in me the notion that a woman's hair is her crowning glory, that no matter how elegant an outfit, if a woman's hair is not right, she might as well get dressed in curlers and flannel pj's. I added nails to that mantra. To me, the only thing uglier than ragged, chipped nails on a woman is a woman with tacky hair and ragged, chipped nails. I made up my mind to go see Doc, prepared to give back those damn estrogen pills and call her a quack to her face.

I got only as far as the receptionist's desk with my anger and bad attitude.

"Trudy, I have been taking estrogen and eating right, and I still feel like I'm falling apart." I slammed the pill bottle down in front of her. "Doc said that I'd feel better long before I turned into the Goodyear blimp. Well, she lied, and I want to see her right now so that I can tell her that the only thing this stuff has done is regulate my period. And, for me, not having a period was the best part about menopause."

By now I was sweating and choking on my tears. My hands shook and my head hurt. I turned away to collect myself. Doc rushed in, and I can only imagine how I must have appeared to her—sweaty and panting so hard I couldn't speak. ·

Doc took my wrist and felt my pulse and guided me to the exam room. Trudy jumped in to explain to the two sisters sitting in the waiting room, with appointments, why I looked as if I'd lost a marathon race and was butting in ahead of them. They didn't object.

Once in the exam room, Doc felt my throat.

"I believe you have thyroid disease," she said. "Hypothyroidism, to be specific. I can't be sure until we get the results of a blood test to measure your TSH level." (TSH is the abbreviation for thyroid-stimulating hormone.)

She told me that the function of the thyroid is to regulate the body's metabolism. When it's out of whack, so are you—sluggish, irritable, sleepy, and fat. Unless you have hyperthyroidism, that is. Then, according to Doc, you're just the opposite—fidgety, sweaty, and skinny, no matter how much you eat. If you have hyperthyroidism, you feel as though you're about four inches off the ground all the time.

Well, I definitely did not have hyperthyroidism. All I wanted to do was lie down. In fact, I was so lethargic that I had doubled my daily ginseng dosage to gather enough energy to hit the courts for an hour or so. Afterward, I'd sit in front of the television and cash in on the chips.

"The symptoms of thyroid disease can be overlooked in estrogen-deficient women or women your age," Doc said, "because they mimic the symptoms of menopause."

"Wow, a double whammy," I sighed. "It's a wonder I don't jump off a bridge."

"Are you exercising as we discussed?" Doc asked.

"I'm learning to play tennis."

"Learning?
"Yes. I never played before."
"That must be . . ."
"Hard work? Yes, it is." I knew she wanted to say it must be fun. "Especially since I'm tired most of the time."

The blood test confirmed that I had hypothyroidism.
"What exactly causes hypothyroidism?"
I wanted specifics. No more of that nature-has-to-take-its-course bull. That was okay for menopause. But she'd called hypothyroidism a disease, and diseases had causes.

Doc related some theory about autoimmune disorders caused by abnormal antibodies. I knew from high-school biology that antibodies are proteins that find foreign agents in the body and tag them for destruction. The thought that something was wrong with my antibodies frightened the hell out of me. Just what was going on inside my body? After all, Mama's tainted blood transfusion had given her hepatitis C. I thought, if my antibodies are slacking on the job, no telling what or how many diseases I could have contracted.

I was so distracted by my thoughts that I barely heard Doc when she said, "Iodine is the chief component of the thyroid hormones and is essential to their production."
"What?" I said.
"You have an iodine deficiency. That's the primary cause . . ."
"Thank you, Jesus," I prayed.
Wouldn't you know it? I'm allergic to iodine. I'd gotten the allergy diagnosis right after I was married and had given myself a Betadine douche.

According to my mama, a douche right after sex was a good contraceptive. Mama was talking about a gentle vinegar and water douche. However, I'd seen a Betadine douche advertisement in a magazine. I'd thought, what better way to kill the male sperm than with a superior germ killer? Well, whether the douche killed the sperm or not, the vaginal irritation it gave me was so severe I had to go to the hospital. I'll never forget the look of amusement on the nurse's face when she asked me if I was trying to pickle myself. I consciously avoided iodine after that. I don't even use iodized table salt. It was no wonder I had an iodine deficiency.

Yes, to pinpoint the primary cause of my hypothyroidism made me feel a lot better. Still, I wanted to know if there was a cure for this glandular disease.

"To have a thyroid disease is to have a hormone deficiency," Doc informed me. "There's no cure for hormone deficiency, only hormone replacement."

First estrogen replacement, now this. No wonder women going through The Change freak out. Their bodies are losing all their juices.

The bad thing about thyroid hormone replacement treatment, as far as I was concerned, turned out to be a little pill called Levothroid I learned I have to take for the rest of my life. I hated swallowing pills. I still dissolved aspirin in a spoon of soda, same as my mother did for me when I was a kid. The good thing, if there could be a good thing about discovering yet another biological deficiency, is that the fear of cancer wouldn't loom over me every time I ingested the stuff, as it did with estrogen.

I decided to scrap HRT. Estrogen replacement had done nothing for my out-of-whack thyroid. And I hoped that the Levothroid would fare better against the similar symptoms of estrogen loss. Considering the alternative, misery in slow motion, and the added risk of cancer, I was glad to switch prescriptions. That decision turned out to be the least of my transition concerns.

My body's meltdown response to menopause was so reactionary it deleted cool rationality from my decision-making process. I didn't see myself living the rest of my life to the fullest, only sinking into rocker mode, waiting to die. The path ahead scared me. Even when my head and heart said why not live it up, my body cranked out all sorts of negative messages—you're older, slower, fatter, lethargic, and forgetful.

The symptoms of old age were upon me, and I couldn't just tell myself to get over it. My past experiences were of no help. I

Thyroid Disorder: The Great Imitator

Thyroid disease can imitate many illnesses, including major depression, heart disease, arthritis, and even cancer. In addition, the symptoms of an overactive or underactive thyroid gland can simulate many of the complaints commonly seen with estrogen decline in perimenopausal women.

Comparison of Complaints in Hypothyroidism and Estrogen Deficiency

COMPLAINT	HYPOTHYROIDISM	ESTROGEN DEFICIENCY
Fatigue, sluggishness, no energy	Persistent	May wax and wane
Depression	Very persistent	Very persistent
Menstrual change	Irregular to absent	Irregular to absent, until mid-to-late forties
PMS symptoms	Aggravated or initiated	Aggravated or initiated
Decreased sexual desire	Common	Common
Difficulty getting pregnant	Common	Common
Short-term memory loss	Common	Common
Diminished concentration	Common	Occurs in late forties and beyond
Loss of hair	Common	Common
Brittle hair	Common	Sometimes occurs
Dry skin	Common	Common

Comparison of Complaints in Hyperthyroidism and Estrogen Deficiency

COMPLAINT	HYPERTHYROIDISM	ESTROGEN DEFICIENCY
Increased sweating	Common	Similar hot flashes
Scanty menstrual cycle	Common	Common
Irritability and moodiness	Common	Common
Heat intolerance	Common	Common
Insomnia	Common	Common
Heart pounding	Common	Common

Source: Adapted from charts appearing in James E. Huston and L. Darlene Lanka, *Perimenopause: Changes in Women's Health After 35,* second edition (Oakland, CA: New Harbinger Publications, 2001; 800-748-6273; www.newharbinger.com).

couldn't just leave the bad behind. I couldn't quit and start fresh the way I did when I left court reporting to work in corporate America because I didn't see the justice in the criminal court system.

Nonetheless, notwithstanding my hormonal deficiencies and the effect those deficiencies were having on the physical and mental stimulation I got from playing tennis, quitting and settling into a rocker were no longer acceptable options. I'd become a tennis junkie. The more I trained, the more I wanted to train. And it's a good thing I didn't quit, because I learned a lot on the tennis court, not just about the game, but about me.

A game of tennis entails not only hitting the ball over the net, but strategically placing it so that your opponent can't get to it. Not just smashing back a ball that's hit to you, but stroking it with just the right amount of force and finesse so that you, the ball stroker, determine where, how fast, or even if the ball is returned to you. To accomplish this control, a player must be mentally prepared and skilled. She must develop a battle plan and muster the courage to see it through.

Life situations are controlled that way, too, or should be. For every major goal of my life—getting an education, pursuing a career, buying a home, buying a car, to name a few—I first had to figure out what I needed to do to achieve it. That's how I took control and was able to put these things within my grasp.

Well, I wanted to become hot stuff on the courts, and I wanted to survive menopause as a healthy and happy person. But with menopause playing with my head as well as my body, I couldn't figure out what I had to do to get what I wanted.

In hindsight, I understand that there was no way I could win on the courts if I didn't master tennis basics. And I wouldn't ease through menopause if I didn't undergo a personal character assessment. Strangely, now I see how working on each one helped me to accomplish the other.

I'd been playing tennis for a few months. I'd been living for fifty years. Quick thinking and movement on the court had me stumped, and menopause was beating me down physically as well as psychologically. I couldn't hit a definitive offensive shot. I couldn't stop feeling afraid and listless. But I wanted to play tennis. I wanted to live an active, productive senior life.

At this point I wondered who had coined the phrase, "We don't get older, we get better." Not a woman a day over thirty-five, that's for sure. But as hard as it was for me to see it back then, that was my basic goal—to get better. At tennis. At living.

And to get better, I had to go to battle against menopause. I had to get my psyche to match up against human nature. But you need ammunition to go into battle. And my traditional artillery—high energy and confidence—were, thanks to estrogen loss, in short supply. Then I remembered Doc telling me that you don't beat menopause. You get through it. To do that, I had to slap myself with reality and snap out of the trance of fear. I had to step up as a woman and focus on living. I had to find a way, a lifestyle change, to help me put menopause in its place so that I could age successfully.

Tennis, I found, had taken on the role of "lifestyle change." I don't recall that being a knock-on-the-head epiphany, but rather a reality that gradually progressed simply because I continued to do something that gave me personal satisfaction at a time when nothing else did. I fostered new goals and dreams for my tennis performance. As I accomplished them and proved my body and mind capable of tackling new boundaries, getting older began to lose some its frightful magnitude.

However, for the most part, my transformation from a menopausal wimp to a self-assured athlete continued to stall. I hadn't mastered tennis basics well enough to play on a competitive court, and I knew that I wouldn't experience a real sense of achievement until I played competitively. But at this stage of my tennis-playing life, my opponents were Coach Wendell, a hitting wall, and Shirley Hefron, another beginner and the sweetest seventy-year-old woman I'd ever met. In my mind, most women tennis enthusiasts my age had been playing forever. I had to make sure that I was well prepared before I approached them. I had to get better.

To get better at tennis I had to step up as a player and focus. I had to watch that little lime-green ball so hard it looked as big as a basketball, so big I could see its seams when it left my opponent's racket and continue to see them until I hit it. That was the only way I would develop the split-second speed and footwork required to hit a winner or difficult-to-return shot.

This pressure and the constant pattern of learning and adjusting my tennis game added new dimensions to my life. Looking back, I can see how they aided my ability to get through menopause. I wish I could pinpoint the exact moment I understood that tennis had become my weapon against menopause. But how I learned to cope with my aging transition was a process. That process was about as definitive and as vague as a coach's advice to a beginning tennis player that the key to playing winning tennis is to follow the ball.

It's true, following the ball will get you in position to hit it back, but how well? After getting to the ball, your shot will be effective if you . . . Believe me, there are any number of things that *if* refers to, such as: get your racket back early, move to the ball, swing through your hit. The *if* that clicked for me was watch where the ball lands. That way you can see if your opponent has to move forward or back to return hit; or if it goes to her strike zone; or if it's angled enough to get her off balance. For example, if she's returning an out-of-reach shot, you can rush in for the put-away. Where the ball lands on your side of the net also determines where you should move to get a good hit in that same way. In other words, following the ball is the general technique. A specific detail like watching where it lands can make your response effective.

My point is that each new dimension in tennis offers an opportunity to become a better player. No matter how well you make a shot one day, there's always a way to improve on it the next. I'd learned to hit the ball over the net. The challenge then became how to get to that same tennis ball with time enough to really do something with it. And since there was no magic potion to make menopause go away, my new life's challenge had to be to revitalize my soul, which had been demoralized by the fears of inadequacy brought on by impending old age. And once I'd learned how to support the energy of my soul, I could take that work and really do something with it, expanding my consciousness not only to get through menopause but to come out a better person on the other side.

I haven't yet introduced you to Anne Lowry, my doubles coach, but she taught me something that I think expresses how tennis helped me adjust to getting older and better. She said that when you are competing on the court, there are three questions to ask yourself: 1) Where are you on the court? 2) Where do you want to go? 3) How are you going to get there? If you answer these questions, she said, you'll find yourself following and moving to the ball, thereby responding rather than reacting to your opponent, and making your play aggressive.

Menopause forced me to ask myself those very questions about my life. At some point, the on-court self-awareness that Coach Anne instilled in me became part of my overall mental and emotional outlook. To quote my mother when asked how she felt about her diagnosis, "I ain't dead yet, so I'm lookin' to tomorrow same as always."

Thanks to tennis, instead of growing complacent and falling into a passive, "I'm in my do-nothing declining years" attitude, I had tomorrow to explore the unventured territory of an organized sport. I could use the youthful fearlessness that expectation generated to energize me through the second puberty of my life.

I never imagined that a stick-in-the-mud like me would reach age fifty eager to expand her competitive nature. Nor did I believe that I would face the challenge of aging with a perspective that activated rather than deflated my physical sense of well-being.

Remember the words in the hymn "Amazing Grace": *I once was blind, but now I see.* The physical and mental challenges of tennis helped me to see beyond the milestone I'd reached in life, beyond the internal physical changes, beyond the fear of mental illness and death. I knew that I could no longer afford to expend the emotional and physical energy obsessing over gray, static hair, age spots, and my pear-shaped body. In fact, I was chomping at the bit to develop a top-spin lob and to further cultivate a winning game and a fulfilling, active senior life.

5

Mind Over Matter

*If you want to raise your playing bar, you are going to
have to increase your fitness level. Contrary to what
many think, you do not play tennis to get fit.
You get fit to play tennis.*

—COACH WENDELL

I n all of my fifty years, I had never done anything, with the
exception of sex, physical enough to break a sweat. Except for
a short period after my second and last child, Teasha, was
born, I never exercised. But after having given birth with my
thirtieth birthday right around the corner, the extra pounds on
my tummy, thighs, and hips were as stubborn as a toddler going
through the terrible-twos stage. The extra pounds forced me to
do nightly sit-ups, which I hoped would flatten my stomach.
(For some reason, wide hips and a wide butt didn't look as big to
me below a flat stomach.)

But in my new tennis life, when I couldn't return Shirley's
ten-mile-an-hour serves consistently, and my lessons with Coach
Wendell were riddled with netted ground strokes and leaning-
tower-of-Pisa volleys, I realized that it would take more than
tennis to fully actuate muscles that had been asleep in my body
for a lifetime. It was time to admit that I'd reached yet another
plateau on my menopausal journey.

It's funny how learning the game of tennis helped me realize that life is one plateau after another. I'd jumped one hurdle
only to face another. So what if I'd come to terms with the woes

of aging and made a major lifestyle change? I still hadn't run through the victory tape.

"Alice," I said, "if you want to live in slow motion, you should take Prozac rather than play tennis."

When I whined about how stagnant and ineffective I felt on the court, Coach Wendell told me, "If you want to raise your playing bar, you are going to have to increase your fitness level. Contrary to what many think, you don't play tennis to get physically fit. You get physically fit to play tennis."

This was not my idea of encouragement. The thought of exercise didn't give me an adrenaline rush.

"Muscle mass," Coach Wendell went on to say, "is the only thing that can put bounce in the step as well as stop fat in its tracks."

Did this mean that I'd have to have a body like Serena Williams to play this game? Who died and left the sporting world to the fit and sculpted?

"To properly execute your shots," Coach Wendell went on to say, "you have to keep your feet moving throughout each point. And to go the three-set distance without zonking out on the court requires staying power."

Three sets! Are you nuts?

"You have got to develop and maintain strength and stamina."

And here I thought walking around the block to keep the blood pumping just to avoid the "big one" would be enough to get me not only through a match but also through the rest of my life without life support.

Sure, I wanted to age healthily. And I wanted the strength and stamina to play a decent game of tennis, three sets if need be, but could I please do it without the rigor of strenuous exercise? Isn't fifty the age when you're supposed to start to live in moderation? Moderate eating habits. Moderate lovemaking. Surely, moderate exercise, too.

I don't know why the concept of "exercise or perish" threw me. After all, my generation of baby boomers not only made muscle-tight women chic, but also turned exercise and dieting into cash-cow life forms. Now, health enthusiasts can't say enough about the benefits of exercise in both physical and mental health.

Where was I while my peers were uncovering the secret to youthful longevity? I was in the workforce, pissed off at the joggers, spinners, and steppers because they had the inclination, time, money, and, more important, the energy, to do so. Let's face it, in the fitness sense, I was a member of the boomer generation in age only. Tennis was my first attempt at exploring my so-called physical side. But should I have been penalized for that?

Two reasons make the answer "yes." First, because of my fitness level, I was physically handicapped and probably would not develop into a good tennis player. Second, I had no way of knowing how mentally challenged menopause would leave me. Therefore, my mental and physical states contraindicated my becoming a player. After all, the game is both mental and physical, and my mind and body were under attack by menopause. Talk about a mind-body connection.

Speaking of mind-body connections . . . after Coach Wendell broke the news to me about the importance of exercise, I started to pay attention to the fitness fad permeating modern life. I was taken aback to realize that whether it's jump rope or yoga, the objective of exercise these days is to make that so-called mind-body connection, a concept that struck me as new-age spiritual.

Everyone associated with health and fitness nowadays, from aerobics instructors to the expanding number of sports psychologists, seems to have become a major proponent of this mind-body trend. And they are all spreading news of the marriage, even to people who traditionally didn't have time or money to burn on fitness, by using their discipline to illustrate the effectiveness of the concept in their lives.

Along with all the medical and scientific data asserting exercise as half of a life's cure-all (diet being the other half), the mind-body thing just put me off as being too much like self-serving organized religion. As far as I was concerned, there were too many interpretations of a straightforward concept: Exercise is healing both physically and emotionally.

Okay, so perhaps my take on good-health theory was an attempt to justify my failure to embrace exercise. But don't get me wrong, I was indeed intrigued by the reported impact spirituality and positive thinking have on, let's say, fighting cancer or HIV. But to me, exercise didn't have that kind of cosmic effect on health. Perhaps this attitude grew out of my belief that exercise was a chore, a boring chore at that. In any case, what made more sense to me, psychologically speaking, was the confident attitude expounded by Nike and its "just do it" campaign.

Despite my indifference to exercise and the mind-body connection philosophy, it was compelling to find out just how extensive the benefits of exercise actually were. Major benefits include the rejuvenation of aging bones and muscle mass, more energy, and increased self-confidence. These are important for all women, of course, but particularly so for menopausal women. Strong women stay young. (There's actually a national bestseller with that title.) But how do you acquire confidence when authoritative sources change methodology on why, how, and what to do as often as women give birth?

The constant revamping of exercise philosophies—what will and will not work—combined with my "moderate" perspective made me worry that I'd never find an exercise program for the new me: the woman with the expanding pear-shaped body who hated to exercise; the woman who'd exchanged the term "declining years" for "inclining years"; the woman who'd decided that because she hadn't had an athletic past didn't mean she couldn't have an athletic future. The new me didn't want merely to watch women grow strong physically and emotionally because of a sport—she wanted to experience it as well.

To that end, I tried every new exercise trend—TaeBo, yoga, jogging, spinning, boxing, Jazzercise, step aerobics—and followed Jane Fonda, Kathy Smith, Richard Simmons, changing the exercise or video tape whenever boredom set in or my enthusiasm waned. Pretty soon, I understood exactly how Danny Glover felt trying to keep up with Mel Gibson in *Lethal Weapon* when he said, "I'm getting too old for this shit."

I was no longer a spring chicken, but I was not yet ready to give up the action, even though following Jane's, Kathy's, Richard's, and Billy Blanks's exercise moves via video just wasn't cutting it for me. And there was something disheartening about working out in a gym with some teenybopper strutting around with six-pack abs and super-defined quads telling me how many sit-ups I should do.

Anyway, remember the doubles instructor I mentioned earlier, Coach Anne? Her assessment, one day in practice, of a play I'd made gave me new insight.

"You stood still a second too long watching your shot," she said. "That made your movement a half second too late. The delay forced you out of position to hit the ball, so you lost the next point. I know I've told you that the difference between winning and losing in tennis is contingent upon movement. But you cannot expect your body to ready itself and to move if your brain is on hold."

Those remarks illustrate what I believe is fundamental to a mind-body connection. The mind-body connection, in my opinion, has more to do with the natural workings of the brain than anything spiritual. If my brain had been doing its job that day, it would have immediately sent the message to my feet to split-step and move back to center court. It would have told my hands to get my racket up and out in front of me, ready for the next shot. *Voilà*—a mind-body connection.

Despite this revelation, however, the biggest problem I had with exercising was stick-to-itiveness. Trainers and researchers alike suggest that in order to achieve exercise success, you should find a program and stick with it. That's the way to experience an exercise high. Regardless of my motivation to improve in tennis, I couldn't stay focused on fitness long enough to experience anything near exercise euphoria, partly because I measured my success with a ruler instead of a yardstick. The minute I could perform an exercise task five minutes longer than I did when I first started, I declared myself fit enough and slacked off. What I failed to notice during those times was how exercise affected my menopause symptoms.

What I mean is that playing tennis put pride and confidence

back into my estrogen-deficient psyche. Every accomplishment on the court did wonders for my negative menopausal attitude. I was no longer reliving the past in my head but, rather, looking forward to the future. I no longer believed I should check out old-folks homes.

But when I exercised, other things happened. I didn't feel like passing out after I'd been awake for an hour. I could sleep through the night. It didn't take me a month to read ten pages of a novel. And I could stay on the court after my lesson to hit even more tennis balls. Still, I did not get into a fitness groove. And I could not see that when my exercise slacked off, so did my life.

In tennis, a psychological tool to help a player refocus and continue to move on to better play is a technique known as the three Rs: Release, Review, and Reset. Literally, I'd released quite a bit over the past months—my fear of aging, my couch-potato lifestyle, and my sports phobia. Now I had to stop and explore (Review) my antipathy toward working out. Otherwise, exercise gratification would remain unobtainable.

Since there's something absolute about the written word for me, I knew it was time to begin my book quest for fitness knowledge. I needed to have specifics spelled out on the printed page. I had to see in black and white what my exercise goals should be and exactly what I should do to reach them, taking into account my age and my lack of exercise over the years, which I thought would determine how strenuous my workouts should be. So back to the library I went.

The books I found reiterated the message broadcast by many infomercials, commercials, and fitness gurus: The tools necessary to get physically fit are the mind and the body. Herein lay my problem—my mind was telling my body I didn't like to exercise.

By the same token, that same mind told my body that it was great that I played tennis, and the two meshed well together on the court. For example, the tennis ball comes over the net somewhere in my space. My mind tells my feet to move toward it and hit it back somewhere in my opponent's space. Figuring out in a split second where and how to return hit and place the ball is what makes the combination of mental and physical activity like a loving couple.

A tennis game can get every bit as intense as a chess match, and my mind was up for the challenge. As for my body . . . well, let's just say it was physically obvious that a fitness program wouldn't hurt. But the truth of the matter was that the only bond between my mind and body as far as exercise was concerned were my thoughts on how agitated I got because sweat destroyed my hairdo.

But what if my thoughts and movement working together on the tennis court was exactly the figurative mind-body connection I couldn't grasp to get me into the exercise mode? And what if Coach Wendell was right, and I had to get more fit to raise my level of play? That would mean I required an ongoing fitness regimen to enhance my game. If not, then how long would it be before the status quo forced me off the court? Not long, if my body couldn't keep up with my mind.

After all, learning the game does not mean you can play the game.

Take Jennifer Capriati's comeback. A professional child-star tennis player, Capriati ran into the confusion of puberty. It knocked the gas out of her career in its early stages, and she quit. When she grew up, her comeback attempts weren't successful until she got to where she had to decide to get fit or never win a slam or become the number-one player. She got fit, the wins poured in, and she reached number one.

While not a tour player like Capriati, I still had tennis dreams and goals. Could I do what she did and journey within myself in search of the mind-body connection, metaphorical or literal, that I needed to sustain my fitness efforts? Would I ever travel the avenues that would enable me to escape exercise boredom? I simply had to get to a place where my fitness level and my tennis game mattered more than my hairdo, just as Capriati had to get past her teenage rebelliousness. Was this a spiritual undertaking or just a matter of focusing?

I honestly don't know what perturbed me more, the fact that I didn't like to exercise and that it had become pivotal to my living a quality senior life, or that my ability to play tennis could be thwarted if I didn't do something to strengthen my physical being. Either way, I was positive that I would not have had this problem if it weren't for menopause sucking the life out of me, mentally and physically.

A step I took to help me obtain focus on working out was to evaluate the two basic forms of exercise, aerobics and strength training, to determine which better suited my needs as well as my personality. Personalization, I hoped, would simplify the process for me and take away my mental block against exercise.

Why I thought I could do one form of exercise instead of the other is beyond me, because I soon discovered that aerobics and strength training are both necessary components of an exercise program, along with stretching. To get fit, I had to do all three—aerobics to burn calories and increase lung and heart fitness; strength or resistance training to improve endurance and flexibility; and stretching to enhance body awareness and coordination, and to sharpen mental focus. In my mind, unfortunately, this was too much exercise for the moderate standard I'd set for myself.

Take strength training, for example. I felt like the pro Martina Hingis, who reportedly took issue with beefing up. I didn't want my muscles bulging like Arnold Schwarzenegger's. I learned, however, that strength training improves balance and energy and prevents osteoporosis (loss of bone mass) as well. Of course I needed balance and energy to play tennis. And Lord knows, osteoporosis would put me into a rocker as well as stir my mother's wrath from the grave. I can still feel the pressure of her thumbs digging into my shoulders as she yanked me upright every time she saw me hunched over.

"God gave you long legs to stand tall on. Be proud and stand up straight," she'd say.

What exercises, then, could I do to awaken and strengthen my muscles as well as stimulate my sense of well-being without making me look as if I belonged on the cover of a bodybuilding magazine?

Since tennis was the reason for my getting into this physical fitness foray, I read up on tennis fitness requirements for the answer. I figured that if I knew precisely what exercises Coach Wendell referred to when he told me that players get fit to play tennis, and not the other way around, my mind might be more inclined to make an exercise connection with my body. In other words, what specific tennis benefit would I get, from say, a bench squat?

For a while I actually did focus on how a particular exercise helped me perform a particular task better on court. For example, to hit a top-spin ground stroke, I had to whip my torso into shape. That meant torso twists, rowing motions, and lunges three times a week, two sets of twelve. But as the number of my tennis tasks increased, so did the number of exercises. Unfortunately, so did boredom.

Next I tried aerobic exercise tapes. From each one, I made a list of what I enjoyed and didn't enjoy doing. For example, TaeBo was too fast, though the kicks and boxing techniques were fun. Richard Simmons lacked even modest intensity, but his music selections were stirring. Jane Fonda and Kathy Smith were paced right, but some of the dance steps were difficult. Not all black people can dance, you know.

I made another list of the differences these methods made on my physicality, either in how I looked or how I felt. For instance, by the time I'd stopped doing TaeBo, I'd lost a few pounds, a few inches around my waist in particular. Kathy left me energized, good to go for almost the entire day. Jane made me feel really good about myself. There's something complimentary in her tone of voice, and I felt pleased with myself after finishing one of her taped sessions. But the monotony got to me. I started skipping my scheduled exercise hour occasionally, and before I realized it, I'd begun to skip it altogether.

As for stretching, I took a yoga class. Mind you, what I knew about yoga came from eavesdropping on a fellow passenger's conversation on a plane ride to New Orleans. This conversation planted the seed in my head that the spiritual connection a person had to make with yoga was too farfetched for me. I couldn't imagine performing her ritual: rising at 5 A.M., relaxing her body like a noodle, then stretching for an hour, day in and day out. However, being the magazine junkie that I am, I'd read in several star publications that Madonna and several other super-svelte celebrities swear that yoga postures stretch the body in a way that soothes and rejuvenates the muscles and the mind. That's what convinced me to give yoga a try.

Soothing and rejuvenating isn't how I'd describe my yoga experience. Painful and demoralizing is more appropriate. I watched my instructor and others in the class twist and stretch their bodies as if they were boneless. Not in a million years would my body bend that way. I was too tight and inflexible. I realize now that the problem was more in my head than with my body. In any case, I didn't go back.

At this point in my tennis-playing life, I had not yet experienced being in the zone, which according to the experts is a mind-body connection so intense that time slows and the game just flows. However, the basic fusion of mental and physical activity that I had experienced on the court did make me aware of the effectiveness of a mind-body connection. To experience being in the zone, or just to get better at tennis, I had to figure out how to get my brain to communicate exercise movement to my body. If not, exercise would always be a boring chore, and my tennis game would not be the best that it could be.

Most of my life, I have done what I had to do with little thought to what I wanted or liked to do. I had to study business in college instead of English, or I wouldn't get the tuition waiver the university I worked for afforded employees. Now I had to exercise in order to *live* the rest of my life. If only I could ignore the fact that I didn't want to stuff my jelly belly into a pair of tights to sweat and grunt for an hour or so every day.

Searching for my ideal exercise regimen led me to read an article on walking. Walking, it said, is cost- and stress-free and, if done three or four times a week, can be an effective total-body workout.

Walking? A total-body workout? What must trainers and gym rats think? They're constantly coming up with other ways to get and stay fit. Could it be that when all else fails, walking has magical exercise powers?

Couldn't prove it by me. Oh, don't scoff at my attitude. Evidently, there are billions, trillions, of people out there who have a hard time buying into the walk-fit franchise. What else justifies why there are so many non-energized, unhealthy people "walking" around?

My high-school civics teacher, Mr. Bottomhiggins, had a heart attack during my junior year. Afterward, he took to walking to and from school, about two miles total in a day. He said it built up his heart muscles. One day, a fellow teacher offered him a ride.

"No, thank you," he said. "Doctor's orders."

The next day it rained, and I saw him hop into that same teacher's car.

Well, my route to school back then was even farther. I walked something like four miles a day, no matter what the weather. I failed to see how it made me more fit. In fact, I did absolutely nothing athletic and barely made it through physical education my entire high-school career. And what about the miles I walked to and from my places of employment? Until I could afford a car, I walked miles to and from bus stops. Sometimes I had to walk from work to my home. Those long hikes didn't do anything but tire me out.

Whether due to avarice or common sense, the flow of articles and books on walking was endless. And they all touted walking as maybe the perfect exercise. One article, written by a female doctor, stated that if everyone in the United States were to walk briskly thirty minutes a day, the incidence of many chronic diseases could be cut by 30 to 40 percent. If this is true, why isn't every able-bodied human being walking briskly for thirty minutes a day? Especially since walking, I read, is ideal for people who aren't always up for a full-blown sweat session. I considered my hair and thought, what a concept for a fitness fickle like me!

But how far and how fast did a sweat-free walker have to walk to reap that full-body workout benefit? Surely, that wasn't the result of a normal gait. Then I finished reading the passage: "Combined with stretches and a couple of days of strength training, brisk walking will increase endurance and burn comparable calories to running."

Therefore, even if I walked briskly for, say, two or three miles, or fifty miles for that matter, swinging my arms and swaying my hips, I still had to do resistance exercises to improve the quality of my life and, thereby, enhance my tennis game.

One thing I learned from playing tennis was that I liked being outside. Outside activity had gotten me off the couch, moving and feeling good about myself. Therefore, I began taking walks for my aerobic exercise.

Also, I rationalized that, since I'm at high risk for cancer and diabetes, and since my youngest brother died from heart failure at age forty-six, and since walking is supposed to be stress-free, what harm would it do me to get with a walk-fit program? Aside from that, walking worked for me psychologically. It didn't offend my ego. I didn't have to prove anything to any muscle-bulging trainer or expose my fat rolls in some cutesy exercise outfit.

Unfortunately, however, the only euphoric experience I had while walking was reveling in the California landscape. This was not a bad thing. At least it kept me walking. Then rainy season began, and more often than not, the walking trails were rained out. But the bad news was that the treadmill just didn't sustain my fitness effort. I guess I needed the trails and landscape to make walking more like fun than exercising. And without tennis—the courts were also rained out—all I needed was an excuse not to exercise. I'd tell myself that I couldn't play, so why work out?

How sad was it that I hated to exercise so much I couldn't stick with a simple walking regimen? My self-esteem took another nosedive.

It was time to shift gears, to "Reset," but to what? I'd ignored my physical side for so many years, I had no history on which to reflect and/or use as a basis to reenergize. Not even my need to avoid disease had had an impact. The only thing that had motivated me to get fit was my desire to play tennis. Once again, I had to use the game to engage my body in exercise, which was, as my new sporting life dictated, a very important component to successful aging.

If Mama had been around, she would've said, "Exercise has to be your means to an end."

Since I always had to force myself to exercise, and my tennis game was dragging and sagging because I wasn't fit enough to challenge myself more on the court, I decided to reevaluate the components of an exercise regimen. Perhaps exercising wouldn't be such a bore and chore if I could eliminate whatever I didn't like without sacrificing efficiency. I asked, What constant activity is woven through each facet of exercise that enhances its effectiveness? I was looking for something so straightforward and so simple that it had gotten lost in interpretations of all the exercise-for-good-health rhetoric.

Two things emerged: Pay strict attention to form, and breathe.

I could understand form. I'd bent over from the waist to pick up a newspaper one day and ended up with a sciatic nerve problem and a backache that literally floored me. But breathing, on the other hand, is natural, I thought. Why the emphasis on that?

According to the written sources, proper breathing during exercise steps up metabolism and tones the abdominal area. Further, breathing uses muscles that reduce tension and anxiety. This sounded good to me, especially since my jelly belly and my constant state of anxiety were telling and problematic areas for me in my menopausal state.

Since yoga is based on the principles of breath and motion, I decided to revisit the practice, but this time with an open mind. Hard as I tried, though, I couldn't relax like a noodle. And for the life of me, I couldn't get my body to bend without pain.

After I missed several pre-paid sessions, even though I hated to waste money, the instructor called me. I told her about my aversion to yoga. She suggested I take up Pilates instead.

She said, "Even though Pilates conditioning is like yoga, with emphasis on deep breathing and mind-body-type methods of motion, the Pilates process is more . . . more . . . how should I say it? More like calisthenics. More external."

External, huh? Well, I wasn't getting anywhere with the internal stuff, that's for sure.

"Isn't some type of expensive equipment needed to do Pilates?" I asked. I didn't want to fill my garage with useless exercise gadgets and equipment.

"Yes," she said. "But that's not what I'm advocating for you at this time. There's a very effective Pilates mat series I'm sure will work for you. You're a tennis player, aren't you?"

"Yes," I said, smiling. I liked the sound of "You're a tennis player."

"Well, Pilates was designed to provide support and strength to the spine by developing the muscles in the body's core that . . ."

"The body's core?"

"Yes, the abdomen, lower back, and buttocks. It's referred to as the 'powerhouse' in the practice of Pilates, and the 'trunk' in tennis."

Powerhouse, huh? It's the fat-storage house when menopause sets in.

"Didn't you know," she asked, "that a strong trunk is the force behind great tennis shots like the forehand, the backhand swing, even the overhead?"

I recalled tennis instructions like "let your knees face the net and turn your trunk" to hit through a ground stroke or to give punch to the volley. Coach Anne had told me that tennis appears to be an upper-body sport but actually starts at the ground level and works its way up to the waist (the powerhouse). She'd said time and again that a tennis player should have strong abs, because strong abs protect the back.

Could this specific promise to strengthen my body's core to become a tennis powerhouse be the connection my mind and body needed to get me up for exercising?

If I broke my legs, I could still walk with crutches or a walker. But if I broke my back, my legs wouldn't budge. Should I concentrate on how to acquire strong abs and a strong back as a way of focusing on exercising? I thought, clearly this is as good an exercise motivator as I was going to get, at least until I had that in-the-zone experience to call upon.

I was right, because my mind and body came together a hell of a lot easier with technical instructions—hug your knees, keep chin to chest, inhale rolling back, and exhale rolling forward (the Pilates exercise called rolling like a ball)—than with metaphorical instructions like "relax like a noodle."

Furthermore, there's no need to burn and sweat to see and feel the results of Pilates. A few spine stretches done exactly right—abdomen flat, arms raised overhead, inhale, chin to chest, roll up, exhale, stretch forward, inhale, roll back, exhale—are as effective, maybe even more so, than beaucoup sit-ups. Success with Pilates comes with regularity and quality of motion, not quantity.

Pilates offered me that same sense of challenge and accomplishment I got when I played tennis. No matter how good my forehand got, I was constantly being shown ways to tweak its effectiveness. Likewise, even though there are specific positions to learn in the basic Pilates mat series, a motion can always be added to up the ante, like lowering the legs to intensify leg stretching.

Was this an example of a mind-body connection? It was to me. After only a few exercises in a Pilates mat session, such as the spine stretch, leg circles, and rolling like a ball, I felt good. I was energetic, my thoughts were clearer, and I was eager to smile. I ask, how cosmic was that?

Another exercise tool that works for me is music. I've always loved music, but I have to admit that I've never had rhythm, not the natural rhythm that's supposed to be innate in black people. The lack of this cultural gene affected my timing on the court. Even though I could get to a ball to hit it, I would either run into it, or I would stop so far away that I'd have to stretch as far as I could to get my racket on it. As a result, I was the most overworked player on the court. That is, until Coach Anne explained the rhythm of the game to me.

It goes like this: *bounce-hit.* In other words, set up (turn, bend knees, and get racket back) when the ball bounces. Then follow through (bring the racket inclining upward to the shoulders, kissing the chin) when you strike the ball. Until these motions become second nature, Coach Anne told me, sing the words *bounce-hit* as you perform the ball stroke. I couldn't believe how much time I had to hit and recover after each shot once I got into that rhythm. What a thrill it gave me to get to a ball in time to hit it well, with power and good placement.

Music provided me the means to use that rhythm-of-the-game approach for inspiration during my exercise regimen. Whether it was the beat from breathing during Pilates postures (inhale for five counts, exhale for five counts) or the beat of tunes from a recording I listened to while walking, music (rhythm) added the adrenaline rush I needed to pursue exercising.

I like Motown sixties and seventies music, which, in my opinion, is the sound track to baby-boomer sagas all over the world. It's the music of my youth, and hearing it sends me back to a time when moving around and exerting my body was not only exhilarating but loads of fun. There's nothing more rejuvenating than a brisk walk with a Motown CD orchestrating my stride. Leg circles are not nearly as boring when Gladys Knight and the Pips symphonize my inhales and exhales with their musical beat. Music energizes by "youthfulnizing," and that takes the chore as well as the bore out of exercising.

Think about it. Even if Beethoven's String Quartet No. 5 is your favorite music, if it's music that really gets to your soul, it'll get you moving. Just imagine the upper-body workout you can get pretending to conduct the orchestra.

The trick is not to freak out when people look at you as if you're nuts, walking along wearing earphones, swinging your arms in the air or performing a too loud karaoke. I'll never forget the morning Aretha and I hit a high note together on a trail I was walking and an approaching five-foot-tall dog howled with fear.

Once I had my foundation of walking and Pilates in place and I'd pinpointed my constants of form, breathing, and music, I connected them to my resolve to keep my tennis core muscles strong. This not only helped me stay up for exercising but also determined what exercises I should do.

To develop my forehand volley, for example, I needed good

trunk rotation. The muscles involved are the obliques and the spinal erectors. The Pilates exercises I use to train those muscles are the mat crisscross and the spine stretch. Then there are sit-ups and torso twists with a medicine ball.

Knee and hip extensions are needed for serves and over-heads. The muscles involved are the quadriceps and glutes. The Pilates exercises I do to strengthen these muscles are those in the sidekick series, or leg lifts with ankle weights. To increase my stamina, I include spurts of sprinting and power strides by lis-tening to fast-beat tunes during my walking workout.

Needless to say, I'm always on the lookout for different and new techniques to enhance my core regimen, not only because they enhance my tennis performance, but also because they aid in the prevention of osteoporosis and heart failure and help control blood pressure and cholesterol levels.

I am aware, however, that if not for tennis, I might not have figured out how invaluable exercise is and the role it plays in helping me sleep better, think better, and look better—to feel right in my skin.

Tennis gave me the courage to pay the toll of aging: exercise. It fused my mind and body into an ongoing state of readiness, instilled in me an eagerness to get better as I aged, and contin-ues to keep me moving healthily and happily along the path of my new life. What a way to offset the physical and emotional meltdown of menopause!

6

The Old-Age-Spread Impact

*When you have inner beauty, you like yourself.
And when you like yourself, you got the key to the world.*

—MY MAMA

I t's been documented that women gain weight during their transitional years and that weight gain is even greater after menopause. So you see, there's something to the "myth" that the older you get, the fatter you get. How else can you explain going to bed one night a size 10 and waking up the next morning a size 14 and shaped like a pear?

In my case, there's also the fact that I come from a long line of tall, heavy-set women. And you know what they say: "When age and fat genes mix, the result can be something humongous." Besides, as culture would dictate in my hometown, being thin is okay, even expected, when you're young, but a skinny mature woman is considered sickly or abnormal. By these standards, I figured that as long as I could fit comfortably into a Southwest Airlines seat, I was damn near anorexic. In a you-are-what-you-are kind of way, this notion helped me come to terms with the big-babe, golden-girl phase of life I'd entered.

What *did* bug me about my weight, however, was that I couldn't kick tennis butt if I couldn't get to the ball quick enough. Excess weight slows a body down.

Thinking back, I doubt if even God could have predicted this worry of mine, considering the nonathlete I had always been. But there I was, twenty pounds or so overweight and addicted to tennis, the game of inches. The millisecond I lost trying to jump-start my feet and move my body invariably lost me points. But like I said, my despair wasn't about being overweight, per se. It was about moving too slowly on the court. It was about bending the knees to scoop up a low shot without needing a crane to straighten up.

Faced with this new obstacle—or this old one come to light—it became clear to me that, just as the mind and body had to connect so that I could fully reap the benefits of exercise, diet and exercise had to marry before I would become physically fit. To exercise without diet, as I had done, merely toned up the fat. And the weigh-in told the story, made me want to toss that this-can't-be-right! scale into the trash. By the same token, I learned enough about my changing physiology to know that dieting without exercise would do nothing for hanging, sagging flesh.

So, if I was going to become the fittest, or even a moderately fit, fifty-plus player on the courts, I had to come up with a weight-reduction plan to go along with my exercise regimen.

The first dilemma I faced was determining whether or not I was too set in my ways to become what I call a health-food nut. Why was this an issue? First of all, I know people who have taken eating correctly far beyond food consciousness all the way to the politically correct nuthouse. As far as I'm concerned, taking anything to the extreme is out and out craziness.

Second, I'm from New Orleans, where food is the foundation of the culture. The mixture of African, Caribbean, French, and Spanish foods makes my birthplace one of the eating capitals of the world. Wouldn't you know that that eating culture was like a monkey wrench unscrewing my good intentions?

Giving up what I called "real food" was no easy task. Progress one day was obliterated by backsliding the next. My slips into tastier bad habits were far more frequent than my bouts of eating consciousness; they also lasted longer as time went on. I thought I'd never adjust to the low-fat, low-carb sensible eating plan dietitians and nutritionists recommend for healthy aging.

In a typical New Orleans nonprogressive mindset, I had a

hard time ditching the notion that the popular television chef Emeril touts worldwide: "Pork fat rules." Deep-fried chicken, creamy macaroni and cheese, rich gravy, and buttered candy yams were all on the same Sunday menu. Damn good foods, but they definitely would not be considered sensible eating, not for a waning metabolism and not the way I'd learned to prepare them.

The other problem I had in grasping a sensible-eating life-style was that there were as many takes on what "sensible" meant as there were experts on the subject. Jenny Craig. Weight Watchers (the best, in my opinion). Overeaters Anonymous. Dr. So and So's high-protein diet. Health guru what's-her-name's low-carbohydrate diet. The juice diet. The water diet. The six-meals-a-day diet. The high-energy, low-fat diet. The list is endless.

As I struggled to sort through all of the fat-freeing options as well as to get past my Crisco mentality, I was forced once again to deal with a physical aging issue from a psychological point of view, or from the inside out. How apropos, since according to Mama, "When you have inner beauty, you like yourself. And when you like yourself, you got the key to the world."

Looking back on all of this, I can see clearly that, despite my mother's and grandmother's fears and conservative views on femininity, their advice guided me through the anguish of my age transformation.

Perhaps the most significant life lesson I had learned from my menopause experience to date had been how to grow more confident and eager for life through introspection—how to step back and take an honest, realistic appraisal of myself; to ask myself where I've been and where I wanted to go. In this instance, I found myself contemplating the saying, "You are what you eat," asking how these words *did* and *would* play out in the skit that's my life.

When did my weight become a problem? Of course I wanted to blame my added blubber on estrogen deficiency and an underactive thyroid, but could my lifelong habits be responsible? Over the years, I ate a lot of everything and didn't gain a pound, the result of a healthy metabolism, I suppose. But could that past behavior be the root of the stubborn fat on my body now?

With menopause screwing around with my metabolism as well as my ability to reason, it was easier to believe that the change in my weight was due to nature and getting older. That is, until I read an article on stress and comfort foods. Then I shifted my perspective and blamed stress for my extra pounds— a logical conclusion, if you ask me. I ate more, sweets mostly, whenever something in my life wasn't right and I was having a hard time coping.

As much as I hated to admit to ever being emotionally weakened, and thereby comfort-food vulnerable, I had to acknowledge that food had been an outlet for stress most of my life. And to say that menopause had me stressed out was an understatement. It was no wonder I blew up when my time to "change" rolled around.

I wanted to blame anything except what I knew in my heart to be true, what Mama and Gramma Fun, my college Psych 101 class, and my life experiences taught me: If eating was my overriding coping strategy for stress, no diet or wonder pill would keep me from shoveling food down my throat. Regardless of biological changes or situational stressors, overeating was the result of my own choices and behavior. I couldn't blame it on anyone or anything else.

What was it my Gramma Fun used to say about self-control and personal responsibility? Take the time I let my friend Betty talk me into walking out of the neighborhood drugstore with a *True Romance* magazine without paying. Mr. Hillthorn, the owner, caught me and brought me home. I told Gramma Fun that Betty made me do it.

Gramma Fun put her pipe on the living-room mantel between her picture of Jesus and a newspaper photo of Martin Luther King, Jr. She pulled her deceased daddy's old belt strap (buckle-less, thank God) off the nail where it hung by the kitchen door, and said, "You the only one who can say what you can and cannot do." Then she gave me a thrashing that forever took away my urge to shoplift.

According to psychologists and other medical experts, lost self-esteem is usually the result when eating takes on the role of comforter. The experts also suggest that only the desire to regain lost self-esteem, to rekindle self-confidence, can conquer a woman's urge to overeat or undereat. In other words, when a woman feels out of touch with her soul or feels that she's lost control over her life, only she can make the reconnection.

In my case, the fear of getting old, fat, and sick with some debilitating disease levitated over me like a mishit tennis ball suspended in the air. Now, if I were on the tennis court looking at that high ball, I couldn't just stand there if I wanted to win the point. And as fearful as I was of getting fatter and sicker and dying, I couldn't just gravitate to the rocker with my Rocky Road ice cream and wait for the inevitable, either. I had to reconnect with my inner strength and fight to eliminate those fears.

I know what you're thinking. And I have to say that I agree. Sometimes a die-hard wannabe tennis player like me tends to make too much of the parallels between the game of tennis and real life. I admit that I sometimes go overboard trying to make my life fit into the tennis glove. But that was not the case when I decided to unburden my mind and body of the extra weight. Tennis really did help me find a way to do it.

Let me explain. The best way to handle a high ball on the tennis court is to run toward it and attack. If you wait until it gets to you, you might not have the power to put it away for a winner. And any self-respecting tennis player knows that it's sacrilegious not to put away a high ball.

As it turned out, my time on the court was the only time the awareness of my mortality didn't freak me out. When I played tennis, my mind and body connected in such a way that I was comfortable enough in my own skin to feel capable and useful again.

Take the process Coach Wendell took me through in order to teach me to serve. A good serve in tennis is crucial to a player's winning an offensive game. Watch the Williams sisters play, and you'll see what I'm talking about. Since I was a fifty-year-old athletic novice and had to be manufactured into a tennis player,

Coach Wendell put my serve on the assembly line and taught me one facet at a time.

First, we worked on the ball toss. If the ball toss isn't out front and high enough, the body can't accelerate properly through the hit, and the serve is short and slow, an easy-to-return shot for the person on the other side of the net. Then we worked on my reach, that is, how high to extend my arm up to comfortably hit the ball in the center of the racket. Next was body motion, bending the knees and stretching up to hit the tossed ball. Then we focused on spin, brushing the ball with the racket during the hit to give it speed and depth. Deep serves can be hard to return. Finally, we worked on placement. A well-placed serve that forces the opponent out of her hitting comfort zone is also often a difficult shot to return.

It was as though my life underwent a renaissance every time I succeeded in one of these tasks. The sense of accomplishment I felt fed me back my self-esteem. I told myself, "I can do this." And with each success, the fear of impending rocker-readiness ceased to overwhelm me.

But when I reached the weight-issue plateau, my insecurity flared up, especially since the added pounds affected my performance on the tennis court—not to mention the health implications I couldn't ignore. When it comes right down to it, weight and good physical and emotional health go hand in hand.

When this concept penetrated my psyche, I realized that I couldn't afford to do nothing about the pounds I'd gained or could gain. Not only would the quality of my tennis game suffer, but so would the quality of my life, the condition of my heart, blood pressure, and cholesterol, and my mental stability.

If I didn't want to settle into the rocker—which I certainly didn't, now that I had tennis flowing through my veins—I had to attack my weight as I would a high ball. But to attack the fat wasn't enough. I had to make some serious changes in what I ate as well as how much I ate. Once again my mind and body didn't connect. Knowing what I had to do and doing it had not reached the same level in my brain.

Then one day while instructing me on how to volley, Coach Wendell said, "Net play is crucial to playing winning tennis."

How could he say that, I thought, when every single volley I hit went into the net or outside the court lines?

"I hate playing the net," I whined.

"Too bad," he said, "because with your wingspan, you could be a great net player."

He was referring to my long arms and legs, of course. I've since heard Billie Jean King make the same comment about Venus Williams's game.

"Can I make a suggestion?" he said. "Try telling yourself that the volley is your favorite shot. Then watch how eager you get to hit it."

"Nothing is that simple, Coach," I said.

Later, though, remembering his words made me think about the day I'd cried in my Gramma Fun's lap because my hair wasn't yellow. To make a long story short, I'd begged Mama to dye my hair yellow. I was just a kid, about six or so, and going through what a lot of poor black kids went through when they saw happy-go-lucky yellow-haired kids in stores or on television, when their favorite dolls' heads were cluttered with yellow locks. Why, even the hair on our homemade dolls, rope stuffed into Coke bottles with clothespins, was the yellow twine used to wrap cotton bails.

Gramma Fun picked me up, carried me to the bathroom mirror, and made me look.

"See that nappy hair?" she said. "God gave it to you. And God don't make nothin' bad or nothin' he don't love. And He musta thought you was special, 'cause everybody ain't got nappy hair like yours."

Coach Wendell's suggestion that I simply tell myself I liked to volley reminded me that self-love, which can be undermined by the fears of menopause, is a strong motivator. Spurred by my memories and what had transpired on the court, I was forced to reflect on my new life and the future I faced. Menopause had put me into a serious funk. Not only did the emotional symptoms make me crazy, but the physical repercussions continued to affect my new life. And to boot, I had to deal with the shock that time, life, was running out.

I looked into my soul's mirror and examined not just my emotional twists and turns, but also the physical changes brought on by aging: graying hair, dry skin, added weight. And then there was, of course, my new love for tennis to consider. To get through to the other side of discontent, I had to employ Gramma Fun's love-the-one-you're-with concept and exchange the self-loathing lurking around inside of me for a positive desire to feel good about who I had become.

Clarity and perspective on the food/weight issue didn't just happen. In fact, for a while I was on a never-ending hunt for the right diet. Weight Watchers, Jenny Craig, Atkins—you name it, I tried it and ended up on that roller coaster I thought I was too smart to get on. Then, worse yet, Doc told me she was moving away and the clinic was closing.

Doc had prepared a list of what she called "fine women medical practitioners" for me to consider. "They're affiliated with Kaiser, an HMO," she said. "You have to become a member to receive their services. This HMO is the best in the state and is known for its prevention programs."

Doc didn't give me a chance to vent the frustration I know she saw bringing tears to my eyes, but went on to describe the prevention theory, which she thought would work for me given my wary attitude toward doctors. Basically, the prevention theory says that you should keep your body fueled properly and your weight in check to ward off life-threatening illnesses. To me this meant keeping my body medicine-free and out of the hands of doctors, particularly male doctors. As a result, my urge to go on a tirade changed to a plan of action.

My first obligation after joining Kaiser was to select a primary-care physician. I was more than pleased to learn that Doc was right when she'd told me that it was up to me to choose my doctor and decide whether or not that doctor would be male or female. I was afraid that the bureaucracy of the omnipotent insurance carrier would somehow override that freedom.

After I selected a female primary-care physician, I enrolled in a ten-week nutrition class designed to teach patients how eating right prevents heart attacks, strokes, and other ailments. Through this class, I wanted to improve my physical specimen by improving the quality as well as lessening the quantity of my food intake. But the reason I began my health quest with a nutrition class has deeper roots, specifically, the view that when you turn fifty, life-threatening illnesses come to roost like chickens. Despite what Doc had told me and what I'd experienced and learned so far about The Change and its relationship to other sicknesses, deep down I still believed my mother was right, that going through The Change meant knocking at death's door. But unlike Gramma Fun and Grammy Cap (my father's mother), who cooked and ate without a nutritional clue, I'd learned enough to know that I didn't want my body to be either run-down or a poisoned sledgehammer when it neared my time to knock.

In addition, I'd rejected Frank's suggestion that alternative medicine such as acupuncture and Eastern herbology might help my weight problem, as well as some of my other menopause symptoms. Frank, who is obsessed with weight, his and now mine, had had the needles stuck in him often enough and had drunk enough herbal weed-and-seed concoctions to slim down the entire Bay Area population. Nevertheless, his complaints about his aches and pains had not subsided, and as far as I could see, his weight issues remained unchanged.

I hoped that the prevention theory advocated by Western medicine, and the HMO Kaiser in particular, would give me a leg up on illnesses precipitated by bad eating habits and by aging. I figured that once I had full knowledge of those illnesses, and how they related to diet specifically, I would not only extend my life, but also lose the slow-me-down weight I'd gained. On top of that, I'd get Dr. "herbalessence" Frank off my case. I got enough flak from my body. I didn't need to hear from him how aging affected me.

Further, deep down I secretly hoped that losing weight would turn back the clock and give me a shot at perhaps a fraction of Venus Williams-like speed on the court. After all, we did have the same lanky build, or at least we did when I was younger. I came to realize, however, that there's nothing more life-threatening than nostalgia when your future is fused with images of flabby skin, gum disease, and endless hours of staring into space. Retrospectively, I have to admit that my expectations for that nutrition class were . . . well, let's just say that my eyes were bigger than my stomach.

Although I'd jumped into the diet situation expecting to be reborn a thin, energetic person, what I ended up having to do instead was deal with how the pounds had piled on in the first place, notwithstanding the role of estrogen loss, the natural effects of the aging process, and the symptoms of an underactive thyroid. I found myself considering things like a lifetime of movie-going accompanied by eating large tubs of buttered popcorn. And eating gallons of Rocky Road ice cream to nurture bouts of the blues. And driving to the supermarket all of three blocks away. These and other habits added up to a simple truth that proved almost as difficult to own up to as menopause: For too long I had eaten and sat around way too much.

The fact of the matter is that when you hog the couch, the remote, and food, not only can you get fat, but you can also heighten your chances of living a diseased and/or shortened senior life. It's as simple as that. But how difficult is it to grasp anything simple? Sometimes we humans just seem to thrive on complexity and stumble on simplicity. Even in tennis. I can't tell you how many times I've watched a pro player make an impossible hit, and miss the easy shot.

Gramma Fun used to say that it's easy to do the wrong thing, but it takes true grit to do what's right, which, quite frankly, explains why we do not have world peace. If every person would follow the simple rule to treat others as they would like to be treated, there'd be no wars.

By the same token, simple tasks should require simple solutions. But sometimes, the simpler the remedy, the more difficult it is to pull off. Gramma Fun used to say, "If somethin' is worth havin', you ain't gonna come by it easy."

This philosophy has led me to believe that the reality of

"simple" in this talk-show age of psychoanalysis, surveys, and studies is too often lost in a sea of data and theories. And there's no facet of life more theorized and data-ized than eating and weight. A case in point is the ongoing rhetoric around the macronutrients: proteins, carbohydrates, and fats.

These three macronutrients are the only forms by which we can ingest calories. No matter what television network we watch, radio station we listen to, or newspaper or periodical we read, there's some mention of these macronutrients in relation to health. Carbohydrates do this. Proteins provide that. Fats are responsible for this. And for every mention, there's a theory backed up by a study on how to make them work for a better "you."

For instance, fat has gotten the rap for obesity and degenerative diseases, including heart failure and high blood pressure. If that's our understanding of fats, how confusing is it to accept a study that says a body needs fats to supply essential fatty acids that aid the proper function of the immune system and balance hormones that keep blood sugar levels stabilized to control hunger?

I read in one dietary report that without proteins, we lose muscle mass and the body cannibalizes itself—in order to build and repair bones, nails, skin, hair, blood, brain cells, and hormones, and to help burn fat. How scary is that? But who do you believe when one expert says that a body needs a high-protein diet for energy and another believes that a sensible eating plan limits protein intake?

Some expert or another concluded that all carbohydrates are composed of sugar that can be used in the body as energy or stored as fat. Another study, while it doesn't disagree with that hypothesis, proved that there are good carbs (say bran cereal and oats) and bad carbs (like bagels and potatoes). Good carbs break down slowly into glucose (sugar) and are absorbed into the bloodstream over a longer period of time, so that the body is able to use up more of the glucose they provide. Bad carbs, however, break down quickly, flooding the body with so much glucose that not all of it can be used and some of it is stored—as fat.

Carb issues, anyone? It's no wonder we miss the forest for the trees.

What all that theory and data mumbo jumbo boils down to, however, is that in order to live, humans have to eat proteins, carbohydrates, and fats. Although the relationship that exists between fats, proteins, and carbohydrates is as complex as it is simple, there *is* a simple solution: Don't eat too much of any one of them. Now, how simple, or should I say, how difficult is that? Simple/complex is what I call it.

Another simple/complex concept I found tucked away in all the information I received about food and health at nutrition camp is that good eating habits are not as complicated as food pushers and diet marketers would have us believe. We're not born craving sugar. We're not born with a gut big enough to hold a turkey.

My eight-year-old grandson, Troy, Jr., came to visit over the summer. One day, I found him watching cartoons and nibbling on potato chips. I suggested he eat a rice cake instead, because it was better for him.

"Grammy," he said, "if potato chips are bad for you, why do people sell them to you to eat?"

A simple question? Yes. But I'll be damned if I could think of a simple answer, which I've come to the conclusion is about as simple/complex as the weight issue itself. Just think: All a woman has to do to become overweight is to eat a lot. But in order to get slim again, she has to turn herself inside out to sort the good diets from the bad diets. To decide whether to use this gadget or that gimmick. To figure out the real before-and-after stuff from the unreal, as seen on television and in periodicals. Climbing Mount Everest would probably be easier.

I eased out of the room as if I hadn't heard what Troy, Jr., had asked and went into the kitchen. I saw an empty KFC carton on the counter. It struck me that if I hadn't seen a Cajun-barbecue-chicken commercial on television the night before, that carton would not have been there. Simple/complex? Go figure.

My "simple" reality was that I was overweight, partly because the juices in my body were running out and partly because I wasn't coping. Both had nothing yet everything to do with the simple fact that I ate too much and exercised too little. Unfortunately, though, the daily output of new studies about what to eat and what not to eat made weight control a daunting undertaking.

Hitting a backhand volley was also a difficult undertaking for me. Yet, one day, when I'd netted that shot for forty minutes of my sixty-minute tennis lesson, Coach Wendell broke in to give me a needed reminder.

"Move to the ball and turn your shoulders, Alice," he said. "That's basic stuff. Always remember the basics when you keep missing like that."

I heeded that advice and punched volley winner after volley winner—proof that in tennis, a losing game can be turned around if a player simply reminds herself to go back to basics. To keep it simple.

I decided to apply that back-to-basics principle to my weight issue in order to simplify my assessment of my eating habits and my extra twenty pounds. I did this by tuning in to simple insights like, *Put the fork down between each bite and swallow your food before picking up your fork again.*

When I heard this advice stated at nutrition camp, I pictured my mama sitting across from me at the dinner table.

"Don't eat so fast," she'd say. "You'll stretch your gut and never fill up. And you'll get indigestion."

To think that my mama knew all along that by slowing down the eating process, you give your body a chance to respond to the food you've eaten, so that you can feel fuller on less food. No wonder I was such a skinny child.

And it's no wonder I turned into an overweight middle-aged adult after having developed the "hurry sickness," that is, gobbling down food on the run. Like many women, I picked up this habit during my wonder-woman years, when I had to take care of my kids, home, job, and schooling simultaneously.

Another commonsense technique that resonated with me was to eat off a smaller plate. The logic being, small plate, less food. Some restaurants have adopted the smaller plate, or tapas style, of serving food. And I suppose that's what those prepared Healthy Choice and Weight Watcher meals are all about, too: proportions.

Another simple tip I found helpful with regard to nibbling on fatty and otherwise unhealthy foods is to make them less visible. For example, to avoid snacking on cookies and chips all night, don't buy any. How do I do this? I'd like to tell you that I'm empowered by the just-say-no theory that takes control away from food cravings and restores it to me. But the truth is, I grocery shop from a list and I eat before I go to market. When my stomach is full, I tend not to prowl the store aisles for goodies, and when I do get a late-night craving, I'm either too tired or too lazy to go shopping.

Another really simple aspect of eating healthy, which was difficult for me to turn into a habit, was drinking lots of water. In addition to the recommended eight glasses of water a day, the nutritionist suggested drinking a glass of water a few minutes before eating.

Hey, I thought, Mama used to do that. She'd fix her plate of food after she'd dished up servings for my two brothers and me. Often there wasn't much left. She'd drink a tall glass of water before joining us at the table and another one after we were done eating. I thought she really liked water.

Even with this insight, I preferred Seven-Up and Coke. But after playing tennis for an hour or two, I'd get plenty thirsty, and no other beverage except water was allowed on the courts. Before long, I'd acquired a taste for nature's lifeline, H_2O.

Also, in my previous young and misinformed life, I thought it was dorky to be nutritionally savvy. I have since discovered that age does wonders for opening the mind. I now understand that it's downright smart to know which food supplies what. In the matter of calcium to help prevent osteoporosis, for example, cottage cheese contains less calcium than yogurt or milk. Carrots are a good source of potassium and an excellent body builder. I started to eat cauliflower, which I hated, when I learned that the National Academy of Sciences singled it out as one of the best cancer-preventing foods. This kind of knowledge can provide the courage to make the attitude and behavior changes necessary to ensure sensible eating habits—which brings me to the other back-to-basics revelation of my ten-week stint in nutrition camp.

Remember the food pyramid? No single food supplies all the nutrients a body needs, but a varied diet that includes many different foods from the pyramid's five major food groups can meet nutritional recommendations. I've come to believe that the food pyramid is the foundation of healthy, sensible eating habits, just as keeping your eye on the ball is key to winning a tennis game. It eliminates the questions about which foods are proteins, carbohydrates, or fats, as well as how much of each to eat on a daily basis. That's why one of my goals became to adapt the pyramid's advice to match my nutritional needs and personal tastes. For example, because of my underactive thyroid, instead of 6–11 servings from the bread, cereal, rice, and pasta group, I cut it down to 1–2 servings.

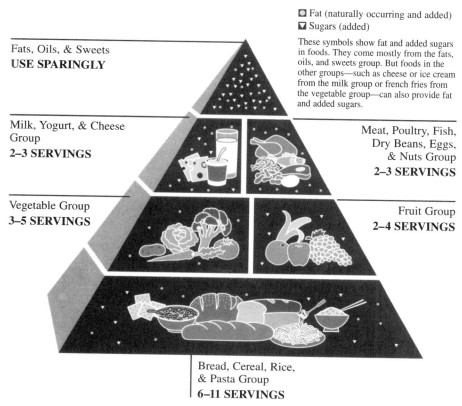

☐ Fat (naturally occurring and added)
☑ Sugars (added)

These symbols show fat and added sugars in foods. They come mostly from the fats, oils, and sweets group. But foods in the other groups—such as cheese or ice cream from the milk group or french fries from the vegetable group—can also provide fat and added sugars.

Fats, Oils, & Sweets
USE SPARINGLY

Milk, Yogurt, & Cheese Group
2–3 SERVINGS

Meat, Poultry, Fish, Dry Beans, Eggs, & Nuts Group
2–3 SERVINGS

Vegetable Group
3–5 SERVINGS

Fruit Group
2–4 SERVINGS

Bread, Cereal, Rice, & Pasta Group
6–11 SERVINGS

Source: U.S. Department of Agriculture/U.S. Department of Health and Human Services

The control-your-weight tip that worked best for me was to start small. By starting small I mean choosing one small change at a time. For instance, I started by putting down the fork between bites while I chewed my food. Before long, I noticed how that made a difference in how much I ate. Then I went on to another change, the smaller plate. I used a Weight Watcher meal container to determine the proportion sizes of my home-cooked meals.

Each little success encouraged and propelled me toward making another small change. Before I knew it, I had made a complete overhaul of my eating habits. The changes have become second nature. I guess that's what is meant by "lifestyle change" as opposed to "going on a diet."

Considering the mental block I had regarding sickness and menopause, food as it relates to illnesses had to come into play. I'd read in any number of menopause titles that starchy foods could homestead on the menopausal woman's stomach. That little tidbit convinced me that the slab of fat that had jellied my belly was the byproduct of estrogen loss, a part of nature over which I had no control. Then my new doctor had a chat with me.

"While the loss of estrogen defies the elasticity in a woman's body, preventing it from tightening, it does not create body fat," she said. "Eating spaghetti seasoned with butter, salt, and pepper three or four times a week does that. And it's the kind of fat that can lead to other health problems including diabetes and heart failure." She informed me that because of my underactive thyroid, I wouldn't metabolize white rice, pastas, and other starchy foods easily. "Combining a sluggish metabolism with the extra pounds menopause naturally adds," she said, "means that you should cut down on eating those foods. Especially since menopausal body fat tends to favor the breast and stomach area."

"Well, alright then," I said. Evidently Doc had noted what I told her about my food preferences and passed those records along to her.

She only lifted her eyebrows at my aggrieved tone.

Studies show that menopausal women should avoid dairy products that are high in saturated fat and salt, which can also affect cholesterol levels and heart function. And I read some-where that a component of cow's milk (tryptophan) increases fatigue. Hell, when my menopause symptoms were full blown, I was a tense mass of flesh in an ongoing state of lethargy. But to give up my blue-day lifeline, ice cream? Well, I'm still working on that issue. Fortunately, some of the low-fat versions on the market are pretty tasty.

One of the most culpable foods during the aging process, however, is sugar. Not only is it hard to process in the estrogen-deficient woman, but it depletes the body's B-complex vitamins and minerals, which can worsen tension and anxiety. When I heard the nutritionist explain this, I thought: Jesus H. Christ. You live fifty years craving a Hershey bar to calm the crazies you get when the monthly cycle throws your hormones out of con-trol, only to find out that when that very hormone is no longer there, eating a Hershey bar can have you climbing the walls.

"That's why it's wise to take a multivitamin," the nutritionist suggested. "One that's designed to offset the menopausal body's nutrient loss. And then there's diabetes to consider. So if you're smart, you'll cut back on the sugar intake. Does anyone in your family have diabetes?"

Here we go again, I thought. The heredity factor. Grammy Cap was diabetic. She used to complain all the time about feel-ing dizzy and spent a good deal of her short life sitting down. One of my clearest memories of Grammy Cap is walking into her kitchen and seeing her leaning her tall, heavy body on the counter, struggling for balance, only for her knees to collapse. She also had to have a foot amputated, and she died three days before she was scheduled to have her leg removed.

I vowed to give up sugar. Not easy, especially since I can't stand that fake-sugar aftertaste.

I'm still struggling with eliminating sugar from my diet, even though I've found that sugar-free cookies and chocolate bars, my favorite, are not all that bad. Sometimes, though, I have to have the real deal. But as time goes by, I find that I get those cravings less and less often.

By the way, I know that none of this is new information. I

have not reinvented the diet-and-health wheel. Like the thirty or so Shakespearean plots that writers employ over and over again, health and diet information is rarely new or surprising. It's the same old, same old—only from different points of view. What I've done is what we boomers are known for: I've made it all about me. I have connected my mind and body via basic health information and my desire to get fit to play tennis. Put into a context that relates to my menopause symptoms, my social and medical history, and my vulnerabilities, this mind-body connection has enabled me to set and reach new goals. It has afforded me a positive attitude with which to embark upon the defining crossroad in my life. And even though I'm headed over the hill to the geriatric Promised Land a size or two larger, I feel good from the inside out. You can, too.

Simple Healthy Eating Habits

1. While eating, put down your fork between bites. Swallow each mouthful before picking up your fork again.

2. To control serving size, eat off a small plate.

3. To avoid bringing home junk food, shop with a list, and eat a meal before going to the market.

4. To control appetite, drink a glass of water before and after meals.

5. Know the basic nutritional breakdown of the foods you're eating. Eat a nutritionally diverse diet.

6. Limit your intake of saturated fats, starchy foods, and processed sugar.

7. To avoid yo-yo dieting, start small. Rather than overhauling your diet all at once, make one small change at a time.

PART THREE

Match

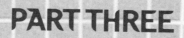

ALICE vs. MENOPAUSE
SCORE: ADVANTAGE—ALICE

Team Tennis Begets Sisterfriendship

Tennis is one of my favorite sports, and my mom's tennis buds reign supreme on and off the courts. You guys make me feel so swell, so please light candle number twelve.

—MY FRIEND ALEX STEUER, AT HER BAT MITZVAH

Team tennis blasted its way into my life the day I met Phillis Lee. I had just finished an exhausting hour practicing my footwork, running from one end of the court to the other, that had left me dog-tired and thirsty. But since my water bottle was empty, I had to stop at the clubhouse for a refill.

"You're Alice Fried, aren't you?"

The sight of the tall, zaftig woman standing in the clubhouse doorway startled me. She had the thickest head of reddish-brown hair I had ever seen.

"And you are?" I asked.

"I'm Phillis, the new manager, and you have to get rated."

The tone of her voice was as commanding as her presence. I inched past her and walked toward the kitchen. The strap on my tennis bag fell from my shoulder, and I dropped my water bottle. Phillis picked it up and handed it to me.

"I what?" I asked.

I couldn't prevent a frown of agitation from creasing my forehead. I reached over the sink and turned on the tap, adjusting my water bottle under the filtered dispenser.

"The USTA season starts soon, and you can't play on the 3.0 team unless you're rated."

Someone told me once that I had an intimidating presence. I'd thought, what a nasty thing to say to a tall woman. But as I stood in the clubhouse kitchen looking squarely into Phillis's brown eyes, feeling intimidated, I understood what that person had meant.

"USTA? 3.0 team? What *are* you talking about?"

"The United States Tennis Association."

I'd heard of it before, but I thought it was a professional players' organization. I wanted to say that, but didn't for fear that I might sound as idiotic as I felt.

Phillis handed me a slip of paper with the time and date of a visual rating by USTA officials at a tennis club in the neighboring town of Moraga.

She's obviously nuts, I thought, appealing to my subconscious to be more assertive. But Phillis looked as if she'd been around the block a few times. A tall black woman in her face might not have the humbling effect on her that it would on some. So I stood there gulping down water, trying to conjure up a sophisticated version of my "projects" attitude.

"I don't understand," I said, more haughtily than I intended.

Phillis's thick brows lifted as if she'd seen me for the first time. I assumed that the flickering I saw in her eyes was contrition. The thought energized my ego.

"I didn't mean to come on so strong," Phillis said. "It's just that there are so many details and so much to do to get ready for the season and . . ."

She reminded me of me trying to get my foot out of my mouth.

"And Coach Wendell said you've been taking lessons for a while. He said you're ready to compete."

Coach Wendell had said that to me, too. In fact, whenever he got a student who played as well or a little better than I did, he gave her my name and telephone number to set up a match. So far, I'd avoided accepting any of those invitations to play. I didn't feel confident that I was ready to test my skills. But he'd never said anything to me about playing on a team.

Aside from the fact that I thought doubles *was* team tennis, I had issues with teamwork. I wasn't a good team player. I found it difficult to plan and make decisions with others. And I'd been forced to be on teams before, and it just seemed like the people I always got teamed up with didn't pull their weight.

For example, when I was in college, I took part in a marketing-class group project. The professor had instructed each of the teams to pull together a campaign for a local beer company, not only for a grade but also to give us exposure to the advertising and marketing world. The company would use the best campaign for one month. There were three deadlines: one for the initial proposal, one for the final draft, and one for sending the campaign proposal to the beer company. The guy on my team responsible for research didn't meet his deadline, which threw copy and art behind. The proposal went in late. Another team won the prize, and I got a "B" instead of an "A" in the course. What really ticked me off was that the people at the beer company didn't get to read the great copy I had written. I viewed that as a missed opportunity, one that I had been banking on.

Back in the clubhouse, Phillis said, "I've arranged for all Chabot members who are not rated to get rated. It'll be fun, and once you're rated, you can play on the 3.0 team. We need at least five more players to fill that roster."

This is one pushy bitch, I thought.

"What roster? What rating?" I tried to sound more put out by her intrusion, which I was, than embarrassed that I didn't have a clue what she was talking about.

"The rating is the USTA's way of making sure you play against players at your level."

That sounded all right to me, given how paranoid I was about not having any tennis experience.

"How does the USTA's rating system work?" I asked.

"The lowest ranking is 1.0," Phillis said. "I believe the highest is something like 6.0 or 7.0. It could be higher. But I think those players have been trained professionally or have played on the college level."

"What's the procedure? What happens at one of these rating sessions? I mean, what do I have to do?"

"You play a game or two while someone from the USTA watches and compares your game play to a specific range of performance guidelines. Once you're rated, you become a USTA member, and you and your rating are placed on a national register. No matter where you go in the United States, you can find someone on your level to play against."

"And the tennis team? What's that all about?" I'd always thought tennis was a one-on-one sport. Frankly, that's what had made it appealing to me.

"The tennis team? That's a group of similarly rated players who take on players, also rated the same, from other clubs and public courts. A team consists of a certain number of players who play five matches a tournament, two singles and three doubles matches. The team that wins the best of the five matches is the winning team."

"I see."

"Listen," Phillis said, "Coach Wendell explained that you're new to the game and everything."

I did not like it that people I didn't know had discussed me behind my back.

"But we thought you'd like the chance to play competitively." Her smile was warmer than I'd expected.

"Can I get rated and not play on a team?" I asked.

"Yes, you can, but at your level, what's the sense?"

I didn't answer her. My mind was racing with thoughts about the new crossroads I'd reached—the people crossroads. I rarely went into the clubhouse, and I never fraternized with the members except for Coach Wendell and Shirley Hefron. Remember her? The seventy-year-old beginner who became my hitting partner? Of course, I knew this had more to do with my game confidence than with any person. I didn't believe I played well enough or that I knew the sport well enough to spend time kibitzing with people I didn't know. I maintained this perspective despite Frank's urging that meeting other people who played would be good for me as well as for my tennis.

I folded the slip of paper and put it in my tennis bag. "Thanks. I'll look into it," I said and headed home.

The sun had just broken through Oakland's gray, late morning clouds, and if Channel 5's Roberta Gonzales's weather prediction was correct, the heat it generated would turn off the Bay Area's natural air conditioner as soon as the sun's rays hit the atmosphere. I wanted to get home before that happened.

Maybe I should get rated, I thought, trudging uphill to my house. I'd been learning the game for months. My rating could not be that bad.

Boy, was I wrong!

First of all, the Moraga Country Club had the homogenized, la-di-da atmosphere I didn't like about the tennis world. Second, I hadn't fully grasped what a rating session would be like, and my apprehension got the better of me. My feet were like lead, and my knees held my legs up like stilts. I ended up with a 1.5 rating, which translated as: still working primarily on getting the ball into play.

I was crushed. All that work, and I'd gone into la-la land and barely gotten the ball into play. I'd been getting the ball into play for months. And I could serve. Return serve. I could volley. Mind you, I couldn't do any of it well, but I had surely gotten past the primary stage. Unfortunately, I didn't demonstrate that to the USTA. Instead, they saw me perform the way I did when I first walked onto the court. They saw me play primary tennis.

After being forced into that humiliating display of gamesmanship at the Moraga Country Club, I wished horrible things would befall that new manager, Phillis Lee. And being too ashamed to face Coach Wendell or Shirley Hefron, I stayed away from the courts. My aging paranoia crept back into my psyche, and I was haunted once again by the notion that I was indeed an old lady. I believed that no matter what my tennis accomplishments had been, I was not, nor would I ever be, a tennis player.

Two weeks passed before Coach Wendell called and asked if I was ill. He said that I had been close to making a major breakthrough in my progress and shouldn't lay off too long if I could help it.

"A breakthrough? With a 1.5 rating? I don't think so."

"Don't let that rating discourage you," he said. "All it means is that you are a beginner."

"But I've been training for almost a year."

"That's nothing, considering the depth of the beginner's range in this game, especially for someone who began at your age and with no natural athletic tendencies. Besides, it takes young potential pros years to get out of the beginner stage. And you mustn't forget that you went out there without any prior game experience."

If that was supposed to make me feel better, it didn't. At the rate I was going, I'd be a hundred years old by the time I reached a 2.5 rating. But I did miss hitting the ball. I missed how good being on the court made me feel. I agreed to take a lesson the next day.

"But that 3.0 tennis team," I told him, "that's out."

After the lesson, I stopped in the clubhouse to, in the words of my granddaughter Jada, "use it" before heading home. I knew Phillis would be there, but I told myself to march straight to the restroom and not look her way.

"Here's Alice now," Phillis said when I opened the clubhouse door.

Had she been waiting for me?

I looked inside and saw a group of women sitting around the lounge.

"Alice, meet your fellow 3.0 teammates."

"3.0 teammates?" I mumbled.

This woman needed a Magnolia Housing Project lesson on how to mind her own business. I'd been rated 1.5. I was sure that Miss Know-It-All knew that.

"Well, actually, everyone is not rated 3.0," Phillis said. "Most are rated lower. But in the USTA, you can play up. You just can't play down. In other words, if you're rated 4.0, you can't play 3.0."

"I see," I said, staring around at the smiling women. There was no smile on my face, however.

I opened my mouth to tell Phillis that if I'd wanted to play a team sport, I would have taken up basketball. Then I thought better of it.

"Here," a Chinese woman said, patting the beige leather sofa next to where she sat, "I saved you a seat."

If I had left at that moment, it would have been not only rude but more humiliating than if I had stayed and just never showed up to play. So I stayed.

"I'm Jane, Jane Yee," the Chinese woman said. "And that's Christina Cory. That's Ann Spanier over there, and you know Phillis."

I wished I didn't.

"Next to her is Hitomi Egashira, Susan Vutz, and that's Jackie McCormick standing beside her."

The thin Japanese girl called Hitomi nodded. Jackie McCormick, sporting a week-at-the-beach tan, and dressed to broker the next corporate merger in an exquisite dark tailored suit, continued to punch into her palm pilot.

The door off the parking lot opened, and several other women came through. Jane introduced me to all of them. Lauretta Brown, a caramel-colored short and compact woman with a flattering boyish haircut, looked to be about my age. So did Jane and Christina, by the way, although I was never good at judging age. The other African American woman, Vanessa Younger, had a youthful freckled face. And Mary Palafox, a beautiful, lanky white girl who moved with the grace of a gazelle, looked as if she'd barely hit the twenty-year mark. Lan Lee, dark-haired, pretty, and of the Asian persuasion, rushed in a few minutes later. She not only looked young but pranced around and giggled liked a teenager. Linda Steuer followed Lan inside. Right off, I pegged Linda as a full-time housewife and mother, and not just because she was accompanied by her two young daughters, Alex and Meredith. She had the nervous energy of an extracurricular activist as well as what I call soccer-mom cool.

While I assessed these women, the room buzzed with chatter. Female chatter like, "Where did you buy that top?" And, "Did you see the hair under Venus's arms when she served?" And, "Girl, did you catch Lifetime's new show *Division*?" Or, "I can't stay long, I have a lot of errands to run." And, "Do you want to grab a beer and some food at Barclay's after this meeting?" And, "I'm busy that day. I have to drive carpool to and from my daughters' swim meet."

I thought, what the hell am I doing here? Mama used to say that nothing but trouble ever came from a bunch of women hanging around together. Hen cliques, she called them. And I must say that every hen clique and practically every sisterfriend relationship I had been involved in ended in some she-said–you-said controversy. Therefore, I'd spent the better part of my adult life avoiding hen cliques.

That's why that day and many days that followed seemed almost surreal. I remember wanting the chitchat to annoy me, but it didn't. I sat silent, frowning, trying to will my negativity into the energy of this brewing sisterhood, but I couldn't. The excuse I searched for, other than my attitude, to get me out the situation never came.

"Okay, ladies," Phillis said, "your first match is tomorrow at the Claremont Country Club. We should all meet here and carpool."

"But we haven't practiced. And we don't have a coach," Jane exclaimed. "And what about a team captain?"

"That will be you," Phillis said. "And I've solved the coach problem as well: Anne Lowry. She can't be here today, but believe me, she's the best, especially at coaching doubles."

"We don't have enough players to play five matches," Christina chided.

"Let me worry about that," Phillis told her. "You just show up tomorrow at eight thirty. The match is scheduled for ten. We'll warm up here, then go to the Claremont."

"I still say we need to be coached before we compete," Jane said.

"I agree," Vanessa said, nodding.

"And we need a specific practice day and time," Linda said. "I have a family to consider."

My thoughts were a whole other matter. I was thinking, could Mama have been wrong about women? And I was thinking that just because Mama had had a bad experience with her girlfriends didn't mean that women who traveled in packs were "back-stabbing, two-timing evil witches," as Mama had described them.

Mama never said why she'd kept her women friends at bay. But her cousin—who I called Tee, short for Auntie, because she and Mama were more like sisters than first cousins—told me all about it.

Tee told me that Mama ran with a group once, that she'd had a best friend, too, a best friend who spent as much time in Mama's house as she did in her own, even after Mama got married. Two years into Mama's marriage to my daddy, she found out that she was pregnant with me. A few weeks later, her buddies, according to Tee, took great pleasure in telling Mama that her best friend was also pregnant and that my daddy was her baby's daddy, too. Truth or not, nobody knows. Mama's best friend left town and never came back. And I don't recall ever seeing my mama hanging out with women other than her co-worker Miss Reeves and the women in the church groups she participated in.

"Don't worry about a coach or anything else." The sound of Phillis's voice brought me back. "We will get to all of that. Right now, we have to establish ourselves as a team, and to do that within the specified time frame means playing at the Claremont Country Club tomorrow."

Who had anointed Phillis Lee the 3.0-team tennis god? And why didn't I tell her how displeased I was at being tricked into joining this arena? Clearly, I wasn't in control of this moment in my life, which no doubt is what I objected to the most.

My emotions regarding this situation wavered in and out of excitement, fear, and annoyance like a drunk driver weaving through traffic on a crowded freeway. I wanted to play. But I wasn't sure about playing on a team. Actually, the thought scared the living daylights out of me. Besides knowing my own limitations when it came to teamwork, I had worked in the corporate world long enough to know how teams really operated—the jealousies, the indecisiveness, the disrespect for ideas and thoughts of others, the inability to follow, the inability to accept an offer of help or advice.

I looked around the room at the other women: Chinese, Mexican, Caucasian, and Japanese. There were two black women other than me, Lauretta and Vanessa, though Vanessa was as light as Linda. I'm from New Orleans where light-skinned blacks are met with the same wariness as whites. And Lauretta's smile never left her face as she agreed with everyone. From my perspective, I was the blackest person in the room, in appearance and in state of mind. It's unfortunate, I know, but more often than not, when a black person runs into a troublesome social situation where she is the minority, she thinks it's because she's black. But even that day, surrounded by a group of women I had never laid eyes on before, I knew that was not the case. I just wanted it to be. That way I wouldn't have to own up to my self-doubt.

I was afraid to play competitive tennis, especially on a team, but more important, I was afraid of the women and how I'd measure up to them. Jane was a lawyer; Christina, a computer whiz; Mary, a corporate manager; Vanessa, a teacher; Hitomi, a Japanese exchange student; Lauretta, a retired manager; Jackie, a bank executive; Lan, an accounting entrepreneur; and Linda, a speech pathologist.

If I had met these women in a corporate office, I would have put on the charm and the boxing gloves and rolled with the punches. But I had never gone to battle in a social setting. These women were at recess, ready to play. And I was in the habit of working through my breaks. Even in high school, I worked on my homework at the lunch table. Not only was I not sure I even faced a battle in this arena, but I wasn't sure I wanted to duke it out, if I had to.

Despite my apprehension, however, I showed up the next morning. I worried about putting my training to the test; about whether or not I was up to the challenge of playing competitive tennis. Also, I worried because somebody else was calling the shots. Phillis had my back up against a wall, yet I didn't blast her for steamrollering me onto the team. I didn't object to her appointing a captain. I didn't insist that we have a coach. And even more significant, I didn't stay home.

The Claremont Country Club was every bit the stereotype the word *tennis* conjures up—a fancy facility complete with women players who donned blond bobbed hairdos and little tennis skirts on their size-six bodies.

We looked like paupers next to our traditionally clad opponents. I wore a black Malcolm X T-shirt and my favorite faded, baggy knee-length shorts. One team member, Alice Sunshine, if my recollection is correct, wore cut-off jeans complete with stylish holes. Nothing matched on any of us, and not one of us had on anything that could remotely be considered tennis wear, except for Jackie's red skirt and white fitted top. That nonconformity to a dress code was part of the charm of the Chabot Racquet Club. But that day at the Claremont Country Club, it was one more thing to make me feel as if I were in over my head.

Phillis had partnered me up with Ann Spanier, a nursing instructor. Ann had white hair and a gentle voice that matched her friendly personality. I was under a lot of self-inflicted pressure and Ann's calm acceptance both of the situation and of me should have relaxed me. But it didn't. In fact, it made me more anxious.

As we approached game time, the skill level that I had fretted over began to matter less to me than all the other stuff I had to contend with. Stuff like the fact that Ann and I were a partnership of strangers. And as if my nervousness about that hadn't tensed me up enough, the wind was blowing out of control. How was I supposed to keep the ball on the court with winds strong enough to push me around? On top of that, I was a little miffed at Ann. All smiles, she didn't appear to be affected by any of it.

As it turned out, Ann and I made a good doubles team. She had previous playing experience and had recently taken up the sport again. Thank God for muscle memory, because when Ann's crosscourt forehand kicked in, it set me up at the net. I grew confident, and hit one put-away volley after another. I had so much fun hitting and missing balls, it didn't matter that we lost.

When the match was over, one of our opponents came up to me. She said, "You could really be good if you took lessons."

At first I felt belittled. Then I got mad. I started to count backward from one hundred, a trick I had learned to switch my anger button to "off." Then I thought, screw tact. This woman needed to learn what my mama and grandma had taught me—that it's not always what you say, but how you say it. Just when I decided to put the woman in the know, Ann spoke up.

"How long did you say you've been playing?" she asked the woman.

"Since junior high school," the woman said, proudly.

"Well," Ann said softly, "my partner started a few months ago. In fact, this is her first match, her first time on the court that hasn't been a lesson. And she did great. Especially since her biggest competition was the wind."

Wow, I thought. The sister had my back!

The "well I never!" look that came across our opponent's crimson face said it all, because she didn't utter a sound.

Ann looked at me and winked, put her racket in her tennis bag, and together we left the court. That was the moment I experienced firsthand what the experts mean when they say, "A good team member comes to the aid of a teammate in need."

I never would have thought that I would experience on a tennis court what I had not experienced in my years in the workplace: players on a productive team sharing not only a goal but a sense of identity, commitment, and empowerment. Further, I never would have imagined that playing on a tennis team would teach me the value of sisterfriendship.

Don't think that I had spent my life entirely friendless. There was Jamell from grade school through high school. My relationship with Faye and Grace took me through college and my first real job. And there was Lena, my best friend, who helped me get through the breakup of my first marriage and those tough early years of single parenthood.

What I'm trying to say is that my friendships, except for my relationship with Lena, did not withstand the trials of my short-comings—shortcomings that I did not perceive until one day not long after I'd joined the tennis team. Someone, not on the team, that I'd hoped would be my friend called to tell me that she could no longer indulge our relationship.

"You are too self-absorbed," she said. "Friendships have to be nurtured, and despite your caring persona, you are not a nur-turing friend."

That stung, but not hard enough to prevent my reactionary response—that a relationship with her would have been too high-maintenance anyway. Thank goodness I was too tongue-tied to say it. I realize now that what she'd said about me was true, and the truth not only hurt but it also scared me, partic-ularly since I found myself thrust onto a tennis team with a group of apparently friend-seeking women. And particularly since I found myself in that same friend-seeking mode.

Funny, but until the day Phillis arranged for me to be on the 3.0 tennis team, I had no idea that a sense of belonging out-side my family unit was the missing part that I needed to get through the rest of my life feeling good about myself. And since then I have come to realize that experiencing loneliness as you get old can be every bit as traumatic as going through puberty as a teenage outsider.

Given the self-reflective frame of mind menopause had put me in, my first inclination upon acknowledging the friends issue was to look back on my past sisterfriendships to determine why they'd failed or why I'd lost contact. But the thought pro-cess was demoralizing. Details were lost in my estrogen-deficient memory, and the absence of rhyme or reason made me feel fool-ish and petty. I decided to look ahead instead. And to prove to myself that I was on the road to sisterhood recovery, I sought and located Grace Thomas, a friend I hadn't seen or spoken to in over twenty years, but who had been as close to me as a sister. Call it a twelve-step maneuver, to make amends. Recovering substance abusers do it to clear the path for better behavior. I guess I wanted to clear the way for better friendships.

Neither Grace nor I could remember why we'd split up. And even though hearing her voice over the telephone made me feel better about myself, I believe that it would have been a wiser move to have come clean with the would-be friend who'd set me straight on the kind of friend that I was. But her issues were much too fresh and painful to confront.

Also, with self-reflection, I absolved my mama of her role in developing my shortcoming. So what if my mama hadn't set an example? She'd responded to circumstances in *her* life. This was my life. I had to hold myself accountable for what had gone wrong in my previous sisterfriendships.

I continued to play on the Chabot Canyon Women's 3.0 USTA tennis team. My concerns about whether or not I could be a good team player continued to grow as well. Nevertheless, my controlling personality emerged. After all, I had spent my adult life convinced that relationships with other women required more emotion and drama than I had the time or the inclination to deal with. But despite my tendency to protect my ego with bossiness and attitude, that conviction no longer prevailed. I'd begun to experience the emotional security gained through social connectedness.

The two things I've always relied on for personal growth are the written word and personal experience. As for teamwork, neither my new experiences nor the written word confirmed Mama's perspective or my lifelong belief of what it's like to be part of a hen clique. Fortunately, the tennis team exposed me to the proper attitude of an effective team player and showed me how a good team is supposed to work. And it was understanding teamwork that helped me realize that I did indeed have what it took to be a team player and a good friend. And it helped me to understand why I had not been these things before. I also discovered that team camaraderie could fill that missing hole in my life. Muhammad Ali, I think, expressed it best when someone asked him to recite a poem after his historical fight in Zaire. He said, "Me. We."

This concept of camaraderie is by no means just my lesson before dying. It is also the result of several studies on aging, including the MacArthur Foundation Study presented in *Successful Aging* by Drs. John W. Rowe and Robert L. Kahn (Pantheon Books, 1998). It states: "Continuing close relationships with others is an important element in successful aging. The mutual exchange of social support that goes on in these relationships has a positive impact on many aspects of physical function as well as mental performance in older age."

Before team tennis, the only relief I had for tired life was ginseng, and I'd come to believe that menopause had made me immune to even that. Now, when I want to feel alive and connected, I have another option: I can set up a tennis match.

One night on the practice court, I was partnered with Christina, another age fifty-plus player. Our opponents were the young guns, Lan and Hitomi. During a play, I went for an angled shot that landed me flat on my behind. Christina, who is usually the one most concerned for safety, disregarded me on the ground and lunged for the ball that I'd missed.

"Get up, Alice," she said. "Get up." She never took her eyes off the ball.

Meanwhile, our younger opponents across the net were too tickled to continue play, and frankly so was I. To see me sprawled on the ground while Christina bounced around like Sugar Ray Leonard waiting for the next shot, yelling at me to get up, was funnier than a scene in an Austin Powers movie.

If I had been the butt of a joke such as that a year or so earlier, before tennis gave me back the confidence menopause had zapped out of me, the humiliation alone would have tortured me. And twenty years ago, when I was really full of myself, I would have been so angry with Christina that I probably would never have spoken to her again. But every time I think about that incident, I smile. I smile because for someone as hard pressed as I've always been to be perfect (at least in everyone else's eyes), to mess up like that and not retreat into stone silence or defensive-aggressive mode was a testament to how team camaraderie had deepened my inner strength.

Later, I read that relationships outside the typical family cir-
cle encourage a person's belief in her abilities. I knew then that
because of tennis, the rest of my life was on the right track, and
I was confident that I would age successfully. I was age fifty-plus
and had been stricken with menopause, but my belief in myself
had already protected me from emotional as well as functional
decline.

Before team tennis, I believed that sharing such things as
hair and nail appointments was just as much a waste of time
as the giddy, teasing, hanging-out time clueless teenagers spent
scouring shopping malls. Why then did I have a blast at the Park
Theater nibbling on pizza and popcorn, watching *Ocean's 11* with
Vanessa, Lan, and Lauretta? How can I explain the fun I had
dancing and singing the night away at Vanessa's surprise birthday party? And I can't express how much I looked forward to the
after-the-match jam sessions where we rehashed our play and
discussed everything from hot flashes to where in the world
Osama bin Laden could possibly be hiding.

I have since learned that avoiding what I thought was a
stressful waste of time brought me only social isolation. If with-
drawing from others, holding in your feelings, and not sharing
yourself can create a murdering, suicidal-like Columbine youth,
imagine then how devastating it can be to an older loner unable
to share that part of her that makes her who she's grown to
become over the years.

I don't mean to imply that I was suicidal or anything that
drastic, but once it became obvious that menopause had set in,
psychologically speaking, I began my descent into rocker-readiness.
I could never have become a complete recluse. After all, my field,
public relations, is a people-oriented profession. And there's also
my family. Still, I was prepared to wait out my time clicking a TV
remote and hanging out with the likes of Walker, the Texas
Ranger, and Ben Matlock, the senior lawyer from Georgia.

Thank God tennis came into my life. While the game itself
provided physical and mental support, the social outgrowth and
my sisterfriendships kept me active and emotionally secure.

What made (and continues to make) my tennis sisterfriendships so potent? So many things. But since my previous sisterfriendships lacked that kind of power, I have to credit the elements of teamwork.

Let me explain. Listening, respect, helping, sharing, and participating are essentials of teamwork. These are also essentials of friendship. Books and journals on teamwork report that productive teams stem from individual players with personal drives and goals who thrive on a shared goal or vision. This is true. Even though I had personal tennis goals, I found it easier to achieve them playing on a team. The thrill of a team win was extremely rewarding, and although the agony of a team defeat could be devastating, the reproach after a personal loss evaporated with a group hug. And although I worked harder learning tennis and played harder on the court, life as a senior citizen became easier.

Sisterfriendships stem from women who, despite their different personalities and points of view, share common interests. Tennis, the shared focal point of my new sisterfriendships, practically forced me to bond with my teammates. The process of learning tasks like how to move on the court or how to construct a point can expose not only individual strengths and talents, but a person's weaknesses as well. How good, then, is a teammate who knows your good points and your bad points and still wants to play with you?

All of the uncertainty I experienced during menopause regarding aging and its effect on my capabilities, as well as how I related to others, were exposed through my behavior on the tennis court. I got down on myself when I didn't catch on as fast as some of my teammates, which manifested as a negative attitude. And I didn't communicate game plans with my doubles partner on court, particularly when we were losing. This failure to communicate is forbidden in team tennis. But I was afraid. Afraid that if I opened up, I'd prove just how bad a team player I really was. Therefore, I came across as self-absorbed.

Whether my teammates saw through my behavior or chose to ignore it, they reassured and encouraged me. I like to think that somehow they recognized my actions for what they really represented—my drive to do well and my need to be in control—and they liked me anyway.

I look back and think how fortunate I was that Vanessa liked me enough to tell me what a spirit buster my attitude could become for the team. Her comment prompted me to take a closer look at myself and to heed a significant teamwork lesson our team's trainer, Coach Anne, had taught us.

She'd said, "The combined efforts and positive attitudes of the players are what make a team work. By the same token, a good team player has only one thing to keep in mind to be effective, and that is, if she sells herself short and isolates herself from the team, the entire team fails."

Studies link social relationships based in physical activity and laughter to longevity and quality of life. By this I suppose the researchers meant that aging women who are physically and mentally passionate about something will not shrivel up and die. Our team practice sessions are a case in point.

First, though, I have to tell you about Anne Lowry, the team's coach. Coach Anne is a gentlewoman with a firm grip on who she is and what she does. But she's a talker, always analogizing to explain how to play the game. Take her spiel on shot selection.

"Different shots," she said, "are like tools in a tool chest. You wouldn't use a hammer to remove a screw. Why then would you hit a drop shot to a player at the net?"

These analogies poured out like water from a faucet. After training with Coach Wendell and his watch-me-and-do-this training method and hearing him mutter little more than "feet, feet, feet" for an hour, Anne's verbosity took some getting used to. But considering my literal mentality, Coach Anne's speeches turned out to be just what I needed to process all that I was learning about the game and my suitability to play it.

Anyway, back to our team practices. Coach Anne started each practice session with a joke. At first, I felt annoyed having to listen to one of her corny jokes every time we practiced. Then I noticed how they lightened things up, even for me. Beginning our practice laughing made it easy to laugh throughout. The laughter decreased my intensity level and helped me to put making mistakes and showing my weaknesses into proper perspective—that is, when learning something new, it's impossible not to mess up. How else could I get better?

Lauretta had a way of swaying backward and making a grunting noise when she messed up a new technique. Not only was this action comical to watch, but the laughter helped me to release the pressure I always felt when tackling a tennis concept or movement I hadn't tried before. Pretty soon, we were all swaying backward and imitating Lauretta's grunt when we made a mistake.

Jane has a distinctive butt wiggle in her serve motion that would fit perfectly into Jim Carrey's animated comedy routine. Imitation of Jane's butt wiggle by another team member (Coach Anne did it best) was hilarious, and it easily relieved the tension when eagerness to do well tightened up task performance during drills.

Mary Palafox, who has an uncanny ability to recall tunes, often broke out in song whenever one of our moves triggered her musical memory. For instance, when Lauretta served Linda a ball so hard and deep that all Linda could do was to step back and let it fly, Mary immediately sang, *"She's got the power,"* her take on the Snap lyric "I've Got the Power." The spontaneity of singing drew laughter from everyone who saw and heard what happened. Especially those, like me, who were familiar with the popular radio tune.

Were Lauretta's grunt, Jane's butt wiggle, Mary's singing, and Coach Anne's jokes silly behavior? I'll say. But they also proved to be valuable tension busters. And according to fitness and sport experts, relaxation enhances learning ability and increases physical task performance.

Also, I found it "youthfulnizing" to be surrounded by silly women, particularly silly younger women. In fact, I'm willing to bet that a study will prove that older women who interact with silly, young women stay young.

The same argument can be applied to interacting with

women from different races, religions, sexual orientation, and cultures. I've discussed how my culture influenced my eating habits. I had no reason to believe that it hadn't influenced my social outlook as well. New Orleans is a hub of cultural differences but it is also a community where like tends to band with like. This separation created complacency steeped in ignorance.

Books rescued me and instilled in me the need to know, while giving me glimpses into worlds and cultures I never would have seen otherwise. In addition, the benefit of higher education that served me best was learning American history, including African American history. Yet, it took more than just knowing the origin of the misconceptions that implant stereotypes to rid them from my psyche. It took confronting them, which is exactly what I had to do on the Chabot Canyon Women's 3.0 Team.

For instance, my notion that lesbians were women who wanted to be men and tried to jump the bones of every woman they met evaporated once I got to know Coach Anne. She's the most girlie girl I've ever met, and a sweet and polite woman to boot, and I learned only by accident, long after we became friends, that she was gay.

I often called Lauretta and Vanessa, born and raised middle-class in California, "bourgeois," because their black experience wasn't the same as mine. Their experience may have been different, but their history is the same, as is the history of all black Americans. We are all the descendants of slaves and slave owners. Their relatives just managed to rise above the oppression a generation or two before mine did.

And my views regarding the lifestyle of the proverbial soccer mom were completely shattered. Linda is certainly not just some wealthy woman living vicariously through her husband and kids. She has her own identity. She's a speech pathologist, an avid reader, a tennis player, and a team leader—and yes, she is the most involved mother and wife I know.

How does interacting with different cultures and ethnicities affect successful aging, aside from helping me shed the weight of ignorance and cynicism? If I've interpreted correctly what the experts have written, I'd have to say that the answer is exposure, exposure, exposure.

The process of meeting new people and learning different things nurtures the spirit and keeps the soul youthful and alive. Think of a before-and-after picture of someone who has lost a ton of weight. Imagine how much easier it must be for that person to get around without the extra pounds. That's what it's like to open a mind to the wonders of human diversity without the extra baggage of misconceptions and half-truths.

Food, like music, is also a great unifier and the best humanitarian around. There is a tradition in team tennis in which the host team feeds the visiting team to replenish the nourishment of exhausted players. This practice proved to be as culture bonding as Thanksgiving dinner is family bonding.

After a year, sometimes even years of separation, miscommunications, and squabbles, families tend to unite at Thanksgiving. I know mine did. Equally, a good time is inevitable for the winners and the losers after a tennis match when there is good food to share. The communication dynamic involved in sharing food accompanied by familial lore not only made our team like a family, but also popularized the team throughout the area for its after-match food spreads and the camaraderie of such a diverse group of women.

On any given game day, our diverse group produced an interesting and tasty after-match menu that could be considered either the cheerleader or the comforter, depending on the perspective of game performance—whether it be a win or a loss. By the same token, the after-match conversations that accompanied those feasts exposed, scrutinized, and put to rest the stereotypical impressions we had about one another. The more we talked, the more we learned about our differences, and the more we learned about one another, the more we tuned in to our similarities. If the world's leaders had conversations like ours, world peace would be a reality.

I'll never forget the evening we all gathered at my house to socialize after a match and to watch the U.S. Open final. Christina had just returned from a business trip to Memphis. She reminded me about the time I had told them that, after the passage of the Voting Rights Act, my local government mandated that new voters compute their birthdays on their voter registration applications. She said that even though her time was limited in Memphis, she felt compelled to visit the National Civil Rights Museum.

"I remembered what you said about going door-to-door to help people in your neighborhood learn to compute their birthdays so that they could register to vote," she said, "and I had to pay my respect."

That's what I call making a social connection.

I've always found it difficult to discuss my problems, especially my mistakes, with others. On the other hand, I could process anger. I guess that was because of the lessons I learned early and often, growing up in a housing project. But it was not easy for me to divulge my inner feelings. Sometimes I felt too ashamed, and sometimes I felt the situation was hopeless and thought, why lay a hopeless situation on someone else?

According to the MacArthur Foundation study on successful aging, older women who bottle up life inside themselves tend to have higher blood pressure than those who are constantly chatting away about themselves. I did not know this when my mama became terminally ill in New Orleans. I spent the better part of three months at her bedside waiting for the end. Two weeks before she passed, my youngest brother, Lloyd, died of heart failure. He was forty-six.

I couldn't have gotten through that sad period without my family. Frank was there. My sister-in-law Vivian was there. My brother, Yasin, and his wife, Elaine, and their kids were there. My sister, Sheila, and her family were there. My cousins, Curtis and Anna, were there. And my children and grandchildren were there. But they were suffering the same pain that I was. And since I'm my mama's firstborn, it was important for me to be strong so that I could console them.

But like menopause, sadness and grief can trigger feelings of self-pity and hopelessness. Also, like menopause, these feelings can defeat a positive spirit if left to fester. Long after my mama's and brother's deaths, the pain of my loss persisted, manifesting itself in recurring bouts of babble about them followed by a flow of tears. Thank goodness this happened in the company of my sisterfriends a few times. Because of the conversations, crying sessions and hugs I shared with these women, I was able to unburden myself of the anger, hurt, and reproach that often prevails after such loss.

Lucky for me, tennis, thereby sisterfriendships, came into my life in time to keep me off the aging fast track. As a result, I experienced the healing power of the care and comfort only special relationships can provide. This significant upshot, or should I say "soul empowerment," defrosted the suffering freezing in me after the deaths of my mama and brother and enabled me to work through my grief.

I liken the experience to having a heart transplant to experiencing an energy surge. The understanding and compassion my sisterfriends gave me, I call a life surge.

Since becoming part of a tennis team, I have worked hard at overcoming my weaknesses as a player. This work, in turn, has strengthened me as a person, although the depth of my sisterfriendship toward my teammates has not yet been tested. There have been no deaths, illness, or crisis for any of them to get through. But I'm not worried, because my sisterfriends have taught me that being there in good times and bad is the glue that holds sisterfriendships together. There is no way I won't be there if any one of them should need me.

Just when I thought I'd reached the age where living had shifted to slow motion, tennis made me feel younger and more alive than I did when I was twenty. And the Chabot Canyon Women's 3.0 Team proved that there is no antiaging tonic more potent than time with the girls.

Perhaps this is because of the women—their personalities, capabilities, and outlooks. How compelling it is to be in the company of women like the ditzy but brilliant Jane Yee, the team's so-called Chinese blond. And the brainy Mexican, Christina Cory.

Strangely enough, Christina is a practical joker as well as the consummate mother hen. Whether she's playing or not, she's always there filling water bottles and making sure her teammates feel supported.

How enlightening it is to share a poem with the beautiful and creative Mary Palafox, a corporate manager with a handshake that makes men quake. How heartwarming it is to be heralded by a teammate's child. I couldn't hold back the tears at young Alex's bat mitzvah when she recognized her mother's tennis teammates as special friends to her and her entire family.

Lan's whiny, naïve persona, as well as her loyalty and devotion, is like a movie viewed over and over. When I'm in her company, I learn something new about humanity and about myself. And the easygoing Lauretta possesses a quality that I'd like to imitate, a quality that understates her passion, at least to a fiery Aries like me: she gives negativity no energy. An attitude like that evokes mental toughness similar to what the champion Venus Williams demonstrates on the pro tour.

And what hen clique or sisterhood is worth its weight in soul without a mess maker? In the Chabot Canyon Women's 3.0 Team, that's Vanessa Younger, dependable and full of spunk. To quote Lauretta, Vanessa is indeed a "shit disturber."

Perhaps what makes my tennis sisterfriendships so potent is their unconditional acceptance of me. As bossy, opinionated, and strong willed as I can be, I never had to pretend to be any other way to fit in, to be liked. But the real proof of the success of my tennis sisterfriendships has to be my willingness to accept them as well as my need for them—emotion, drama, and all.

Linda's thirteen-year-old daughter, Alex, said it best at her bat mitzvah: "Tennis is one of my favorite sports. And my mom's tennis buds reign supreme on and off the courts!"

Afterword

The Reward Ceremony

Team sports is a relatively new phenomenon for women in America. The social benefits, good health habits, and self-confidence it bestows, long integral parts of male development, are now available to women. How lucky for us baby boomers that tennis, the sport for all ages, provides the essentials of team sports—positive state of mind, a will-do attitude, and courage. How lucky we are that these essentials can contribute to helping us survive the mind- and body-altering menopause experience. Not since Billie Jean King beat Bobby Riggs has tennis offered such exciting promise to women.

Take it from me, a nerdy, over-the-hill athletic wimp: Tackling the physical and mental challenges of menopause with an organized team sport such as tennis will transport you from a lonely, slothful geriatric pasture to a "youthfulnized" world of camaraderie, vitality, accomplishment, and fun. Then you'll be able to say, "I'm not getting older, I'm getting better," and feel it!

Appendix A

The Chabot Canyon 3.0 Team's Word-Association Technique and Glossary

Doubles is my favorite tennis game. But doubles is not only quick-moving; it also requires quick thinking. This was an issue for me, because when I started to play the game, I was a menopausal vegetable. And memory loss, a symptom of menopause, threatened that quick-thinking aspect of my game.

Even for the young, with their estrogen-sufficient memories, making simultaneous decisions is tough work. These decisions include snap judgments, such as where you and your partner are on the court; where the ball is; and where you should place the ball, based on your opponent's position.

To this day, it really ticks me off when a lapsed-memory moment during play leaves me standing like a statue holding a racket while I watch the ball whiz by—especially when somewhere in my head is the answer that was put there over and over again by Coach Anne in her doubles clinics. But as I've said, Coach Anne is a talking head in these clinics. I swear, the woman has a story and/or some philosophical explanation to accompany every strategy and technique she teaches. And for any senior player who has trouble remembering the names of her children, sifting through all that garble to get to the nitty-gritty in a split second can be a problem. Why? Because like the body, the mind has to stay in motion on the tennis court.

I must say, though, that from all of Coach Anne's talking, I learned the "why" behind any given game play. For example, returning a shot to your opponent's inside forehand gives her the opportunity to change the direction of the ball, enabling her to hit either into the open court or where you are most off balance. Knowing this, the smart reply would be to return hit to your opponent's backhand or at her feet.

I know that eventually Coach Anne's long, detailed explanations will provide me with the mental ammunition I need to develop a fast-thinking, competitive game. In fact, I can't believe how well I have already learned to strategize and analyze play, even in the pro games that I watch. I must admit, though, that I'm hoping to make an in-the-zone mind-body connection sometime in this life. But, hey, that's what makes this sport a great memory tool. There's always something new to learn and skills to improve upon. Thus the rise of the team term *cha-ching, cha-ching*, the sound of Coach Anne's cash register every time we have to relearn one of her lessons.

I know that I am getting better at playing doubles because of Coach Anne's long explanations. However, my lack of split-second recall remained a hindrance until my teammates and I started using word associations to remember what to do in the heat of fast play.

Say you return a ball while moving into no-man's-land (the area between service line and baseline) and get stuck. If the return ball is over your head while you're in that area, it's going out. Don't hit it. Once in clinic Coach Anne threatened to charge us a dollar for every "out" ball we hit. Thus the origin of the term *dollar ball*.

Terms like *MPB* and *tennis grammy* have more personal origins. MPB (Mary Pierce break) started up when a group of us watched the pro, Mary Pierce, play and noticed the number of times she took to primp on the court: tying her shoe laces, adjusting her ponytail, or fixing her contacts. And when my four-year-old granddaughter, Alyssa, asked if she could take me to her school for show-and-tell so that her classmates could see her "tennis grammy," that term became a part of our vocabulary.

With the long explanations Coach Anne used to teach the game, I had to pick a word or two to assist my memory with keeping a game play in quick-recall mode. Take this example: I tended to stand flat-footed on court while my partner hit the ball. When the ball came to me, I wasn't ready and missed the shot. Then one day in practice, Coach Anne demonstrated how to move my feet and turn my shoulders, and where to hold the racket while I wait for my opportunity to hit the ball. She looked as if she were doing a dance, and *voilà*, we'd discovered the *Chabot shuffle*. When my partner says to me, "Chabot shuffle," I stand on my toes and get in motion, thereby staying in the game, ready to play even when the ball is not hit to me.

For the menopausal tennis player like me, or any tennis player for that matter, word associations can trigger the split-second memory that she needs to call upon while playing the game.

For those of you who have been inspired to buy a racket and get in the game, the following is a short glossary of word-association terms that were derived from Coach Anne's lectures. My teammates and I use them faithfully. By showing you how you can process information about the game quickly, I hope these terms will also help cut down your learning time and speed up your playing time.

bungie: the act of moving with your partner from side to side on the doubles court.

butt shot: a waistline bend instead of stepping forward with a knee bend to reach and hit a ball.

Chabot shuffle: simultaneous shoulder turn and footwork of doubles player while partner is striking the ball.

champagne shot: striking a high ball; or striking a ball overhead while on the run, near or on the baseline, from over the shoulder.

dollar ball: striking an "out" ball.

game rhythm: movement-reminder cantata—player moves while singing "set, through" or "bounce, hit" to help her get into the best position to strike the ball.

gather and go: the idea of setting up for an approach shot to avoid running into the ball and then letting your follow-through pull you forward.

hard eyes: intense focus on the ball during a play.

high hands: keeping hands up and in front, ready for the volley.

hit and hangout: bad habit of striking the ball, then stopping to watch where it lands.

hold the middle: act of doubles partners protecting the middle of the court during a game (like holding the line in football).

hot-flash shots: series of reflex volleys from a player on the spot at the net.

John Wayne tennis: the head-off-at-the-pass play that describes diagonal rather than lateral movement to get to a ball.

MPB: Mary Pierce break; any time used to tie shoes, adjust caps, headbands, or hair, or to remove or put on eyewear.

munchie: the put-away shot of a high ball that's not an overhead.

Oh! Shit–ball: 1) a defensive overhead when you think you've won the point on the shot before; or, 2) a way of alerting your partner that you hit a short lob and she is about to get creamed.

penny point: a missed game point because of an unforced error.

Preparation H: the split-second needed to prepare or get set before striking the ball.

queen wave: motion for turning the hand when striking an overhead or a serve.

scurry: running motion of senior players on court to get to a short or angled shot.

tennis grammy: title given to me by my four-year-old granddaughter and used to describe grandmothers on the team.

vitamin I: ibuprofen or any painkiller taken by senior players before competitive play.

vitamin T: celebratory tit bumps after a team match win.

Appendix B

Tennis Fashion and the Older or Thicker Player

You've probably figured out by now that I can be pretty anal about certain things, and the way I look heads the list. Remember the royal blue bloomer gym shorts we had to wear in high school back in the fifties and sixties? I bet I was the only kid who wore hers ironed. And I got stars on my report card for having the cleanest sneakers and the whitest socks. All this explains why tennis fashion is one of my biggest soapboxes.

Granted I'm older and thicker than other players, but that doesn't mean I shouldn't be able to find tennis clothes that not only fit but are also stylish and compli-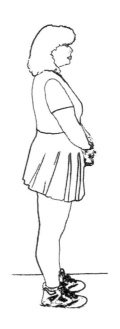mentary to my body shape. And if reading this book gets you off the couch and out on the court, take note of a few fashion tips, because how we look plays a big role in how well we adjust to the advanced aging process.

Examine the picture at right with me and you will see where I'm coming from.

Notice how the skirt is hiked up in the back. Even though it fits around the waist, it's not long enough nor does it have enough material to fit around the butt without spreading the pleats. My advice to anyone with a big-butt figure is, first of all, don't wear pleated skirts.

And if you do, don't wear tennis-pleated skirts. Their size is based on little, short, estrogen-sufficient women. And, I might add, even some little, short, estrogen-deficient women find them ill-fitting. How disappointing, then, for me: a couple of inches shy of six feet tall, metabolism-challenged, with fat inner thighs. I have to wear skirts rather than short pants when I play. Why? Because my inner thighs rub together, and I find it difficult to stay in ready position (holding the racket out in front of the body) when I have to constantly pull the shorts from my behind.

How do I combat that stuffed-into-clothes look, wearing a skirt? And how do I prevent flashing the floppy-flesh jiggle when I move? With casual wear that fits and conceals properly and can be worn as tennis wear. I have found that Lane Bryant's Venezia Jeans brand makes a short skirt that works just fine on the court. The stretch fabric moves and breathes, and the sizes are geared toward the non-anorexic body type.

Once, I found an A-line, flair-bottom short skirt that was perfect: long enough, and roomy yet shapely and handsome. I looked great when I wore it—lean and contained. But these finds are rare. So if you come across one, stock up.

If you have a big ass that's not quite the size of Texas, however, and you insist on wearing a tennis skirt, try wearing it a size or two larger than your normal size. The extra yardage will give the skirt some length as well as eliminate the hiking up around your butt. If it's pleated, make sure that it has drop pleats, and wear the skirt backward. It's been my experience that a fraction more material is allowed for the stomach area rather than the butt area in larger-size, drop-pleated tennis skirts.

Think leopard tennis panties are cute on the over-the-hill butt? Well, think again. Tennis panty briefs should be a fashion no-no for middle-aged players. When menopause sets in and metabolism wanes, the middle area of the body—the abdomen down to the hips and inner thighs—is the first to go fat. If you have fat inner thighs, wide hips, spreading buttocks, and a protruding jelly belly, do not wear tennis briefs. Take it from me, it's a scary courtside sight when you bend over. Wear biker shorts, or short exercise tights, or CourtShorties (form-fitting boxer-type tennis underwear). Your underclothing should creep down to your knees, not up to the crack of your butt. Don't be lured into stuffing yourself into little panty briefs because they come in great colors with fun designs. Paint or sew your own designs on your biker shorts, on your CourtShorty underwear—anything to avoid wide-ass flashing when you stoop to pick up a ball.

The older women I talk to, large and small, want to wear their fitted tops, not have them painted on. Even if she remains size "Brittany Spears," she does not want her clothes glued to her body.

Again, tennis-fashion sizes are off the mark when it comes to mature, older women. Our seasoned fashion outlook and the changes in our physiology are not taken into account. Yes, there are fitted tops you can get over your head if you wear a bra size larger than an "A" cup. But it is not likely that they'll cover what you want them to or what they should, that is, not unless you're the teenage, buxom Serena Williams. You're losing estrogen, and consequently, your body's elasticity. The skin is looser and needs room to breathe. Eddie Bauer makes a cotton tapered T-shirt (tall sizes available) with or without a button-down front that serves this fashion issue handsomely, as does Lane Bryant's Venezia Jeans T-shirt collection. And the colors are fun, too.

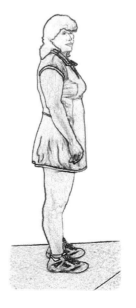

Take it from me, you don't want to look like the poor relations on the tennis court, wearing a too tight, too short, hand-me-down-looking outfit. Avoid the short and/or painted-on fitted top.

What I wouldn't give for a tennis dress that falls a few of inches above my knees with a slight flair, has sleeves and maybe a collar, and shows my curves yet with enough fabric to hide my bulges. Lord, what I wouldn't give for a tennis dress that actually fits!

I realize, though, how much there is to consider in this request—my height (5'11");

my weight (none of your business); my body proportions (larger upper body); and my conservative taste in color. Neon and
hot pink are definitely out. Don't clothiers realize that millions
of bodies and attitudes are out there being transformed by
menopause, bodies belonging to women who will spend billions on sports clothes if they're attractive, figure-flattering, and
affordable?

Sorry, sisterfriends, but the only advice I can give if you are
older than twenty, stand higher than five feet tall, and wear anything larger than a size six, is don't wear tennis dresses. They are
usually sleeveless, which doesn't flatter even the skinniest estrogen-deficient arms. And they are likely to be macro-minis
designed to show off lean, new bodies, not bodies that have
been lived in awhile. When older women wear these dresses,
they expose spider and varicose veins and way too much of
menopause's non-metabolized body fat that tends to hang out
on the butt and hips.

It will be wonderful—and no less significant than Suzanne
Lenglen's daring pioneer move to wear an ankle-length dress on
the court in 1920—when we can find dresses that give taller,
older, and/or larger tennis players like me that Helen Wills
Moody classic classiness on the court. Until then, avoid stuffing
and overexposing. Keep "chic" as well as comfort in the mature
tennis-sporty look.

Appendix C

The Chabot Canyon 3.0 Team's Postgame Kickin'-It Chow

After a competition, the host team is responsible for feeding its guests. The Chabot Canyon Women's 3.0 Team has acquired a reputation in the northern California district for putting out quite a spread. This can be attributed to the ethnic mix of players on the team and the variety of foods they contribute.

As a tribute to my teammates—and as a bonus to you, the reader—I'd like to offer some of the best potluck-style recipes the Chabot Canyon team has concocted.

AUNTIE XOCHITL'S CEVICHE

*Christina's aunt's ceviche hits the spot for
the non-meat-eating "fishetarians."*

YIELD: 8–12 SERVINGS

Approximately 1 pound raw fresh fish

$1/_2$ medium white onion, minced

1 cup juice of Mexican lemons

1 or 2 medium tomatoes

1–2 tablespoons chopped cilantro

3–6 serrano chiles, chopped

Salt, to taste

Day One (day before serving):

1. Finely chop the fish and place in a glass bowl.

2. Mix in the onion and the lemon juice. Use enough juice to cover the fish (slightly soupy).

3. Cover the fish mixture with plastic wrap, leaving no air between the plastic wrap and the fish.

4. Let the lemon, onion, and fish mixture marinate in the refrigerator overnight.

Day Two:

1. Seed and skin (optional) the tomatoes. Chop into small pieces and add to the fish mixture.

2. Add chopped cilantro, chiles, and salt to taste.

3. Cover with plastic wrap, leaving no air between the plastic and the fish.

4. Store in the refrigerator until ready to serve. (The chile flavor will enhance over time.)

Presentation Ideas:

- Place the ceviche in a pretty bowl surrounded with good tortilla chips for dipping.

- Serve as a side to a meal.

- Serve on tostados (crisp fried corn tortillas) with a slice of ripe avocado and red chili sauce.

NEW ORLEANS RED BEANS AND RICE

*Traditionally, Monday is red beans and rice day
in New Orleans.*

YIELD: SERVES SIX PEOPLE

1 pound dry kidney beans

6 cups water

2 pounds link sausage, cut into 1-inch pieces

1 teaspoon salt

$1/2$ teaspoon hot pepper sauce

1 teaspoon Worcestershire sauce

1 onion, chopped

1 clove garlic, minced

3 cups rice, cooked

1. Soak beans in water overnight. Drain.

2. Place drained beans in a large Dutch oven or kettle. Add the remaining ingredients (except rice). Bring to a boil, stirring frequently to prevent sticking.

3. Reduce heat to low and cook slowly for several hours, stirring occasionally. If necessary, add more water if beans are not tender. If you prefer thick gravy, mash a few beans and cook longer. You can also add a pinch of flour as thickener.

4. Serve over rice.

JANE'S LEMON BARS

*These delectable bars are always a winner,
even when the team isn't.*

YIELD: 12–18 BARS

The Pastry

2 cups flour

$1/2$ cup sifted powdered sugar

1 cup butter

The Filling

3 eggs, lightly beaten

$3/4$ cup powdered sugar

3 tablespoons lemon juice

$1/2$ teaspoon grated lemon peel

$2 1/2$ tablespoons flour

$1/4$ teaspoon baking powder

Garnish

Powdered sugar, for coating

1. The Pastry

Combine flour and sugar. Cut butter into flour mixture. Press dough evenly into a 9-by-13-inch baking pan. Bake at 350°F for 15 minutes or until lightly golden.

2. The Filling

Beat eggs with sugar until light-and-fluffy looking. Add lemon juice and lemon peel. Add flour and baking powder. Pour over cooked crust.

3. Bake at 350°F for about 25 minutes.

4. Sift powdered sugar lightly over top when cool, and cut into squares.

JANE'S FRIED WONTONS

*Jane's wontons simply satisfy our traditional
Chinese food expectations.*

YIELD: 12–14 WONTONS

$1/_2$ pound lean ground pork

$1/_2$ pound shrimp (shelled, de-veined,
and coarsely chopped)

4 Chinese dried mushrooms or
fresh shiitake mushrooms, minced

3–4 water chestnuts, minced

1 tablespoon soy sauce

2–3 dashes dry sherry or rice cooking wine

2 teaspoons freshly grated ginger

1 package wonton wrappers

Cooking oil

*Note: Chinese cooks rarely measure ingredients when cooking. If it
looks and smells good, it must be right.*

1. Combine all ingredients, except the wonton wrappers and oil, until blended. Do not overmix.

2. Using chopsticks, place one rounded teaspoon of meat on one corner of a wonton wrapper. (The filled wontons need to be uniform in size so they will cook at the same rate.)

3. Follow the directions on the wonton package for wrapping and folding the wontons.

4. Pour oil to a depth of at least two inches into a large skillet and heat. When the oil is hot, add wontons to oil, a few at a time, and cook until skins are medium golden brown. Cooking time should not exceed 2–3 minutes. Lift out of hot oil and drain on paper towels.

5. Keep the wontons warm in the oven until ready to serve. Serve with sweet and sour sauce (see next recipe).

SWEET AND SOUR SAUCE

*What's a traditional wonton
without traditional sweet and sour sauce?*

YIELD: ABOUT 1 CUP

$\frac{1}{2}$ cup pineapple juice

$\frac{1}{3}$ cup ketchup

$\frac{1}{3}$ cup vinegar

2 tablespoons brown sugar

2 tablespoons cornstarch

1 teaspoon soy sauce

3–4 ginger slices

1. In a medium saucepan, combine pineapple juice, ketchup, vinegar, and brown sugar with cornstarch. Bring to a boil. If mixture needs more thickening, add more cornstarch mixed with water or pineapple juice.

2. Add soy sauce and a few ginger slices. Add more soy sauce if needed for flavoring.

3. Let stand a few minutes to cool. Remove ginger slices before serving with fried wontons.

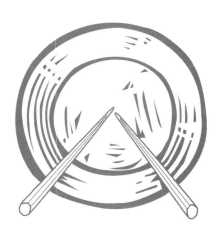

HITOMI'S CHIRASHI SUSHI

This is our good-luck recipe. When Hitomi left to return to Japan, she gave me this recipe and a little rabbit statuette, which was her good-luck charm.

YIELD: 8 SERVINGS

4 cups rice

4 tablespoons sake

8 tablespoons rice vinegar

2 tablespoons plus 2 teaspoons sugar

2 teaspoons plus pinch salt

7 ounces lotus root

2 carrots

6 ounces (177 ml) bonito-based stock

1 tablespoon soy sauce

4 eggs

1. Wash rice and drain for 30 minutes before cooking. Put rice in a rice cooker; pour in water to 4-cup level; take out 4 tablespoons of water and add same quantity of sake. Cook.

2. In a bowl, mix together the rice vinegar, 2 tablespoons of sugar, and 2 teaspoons of salt until dissolved. Set aside.

3. Peel skin of lotus root. Slice thin and cut into bite-sized pieces. Soak in water for 5 minutes.

4. Cut carrots thin and short (about 1 inch).

5. Put lotus root, carrots, bonito-based stock, 2 teaspoons of sugar, soy sauce, and a pinch of salt in a pot. Stir and cook until almost dried.

6. Beat eggs, and scramble in a pan.

7. Pour cooked rice into a big bowl. Add the rice vinegar mixture and mix well, while cooling rice by fanning.

8. Mix in the cooked vegetables and eggs. Serve.

LAN'S GREEN PAPAYA SALAD

Lan's game is always on when it comes to salad.

YIELD: 8–12 SERVINGS

The Salad

1 medium green papaya, peeled, seeded, and julienned

1 medium carrot, peeled and shredded

1 small white onion, thinly sliced

1 small ginger root, peeled and shredded

$\frac{1}{2}$ teaspoon Vietnamese chili-garlic sauce

Garnish

$1\frac{1}{2}$ tablespoons roughly chopped fresh cilantro

1 tablespoon roughly chopped fresh mint

$\frac{1}{4}$ cup chopped peanuts

The Dressing

2 tablespoons fish sauce (preferably Nuoc Mam)

2 tablespoons rice vinegar

1 tablespoon lemon or lime juice

4 tablespoons water

4 tablespoons sugar

1 teaspoon minced garlic

1. Place papaya, carrot, onion, and ginger in a bowl and mix well.

2. Add chili-garlic sauce and toss well.

3. Garnish with cilantro, mint, and peanuts.

4. In a medium bowl, whisk together dressing ingredients until sugar is dissolved. Toss with salad.

COUSIN ANNA'S LAYERED BURRITOS

*Cousin Anna is a cooking-show junkie,
and when I am in a time crunch
she is sure to cook the team something special.
Vanessa sure thinks so.*

YIELD: 8 SERVINGS

1 pound lean ground beef

1 package burrito seasoning

1 cup picante sauce or salsa

1 can refried beans

8 flour or corn tortillas

2 cups shredded Cheddar cheese

1. Brown ground beef. Add burrito seasoning and cook until meat is done.

2. Mix picante sauce or salsa with refried beans.

3. Layer a baking dish with a small amount of beef mixture, then add a layer of tortillas. Spread a layer of beef mixture on top, then add another layer of tortillas. Pour all of the bean mixture on top, followed by another layer of tortillas. Add a layer of cheese and a final layer of tortillas. Spread on the remaining beef mixture and cheese.

4. Bake at 375°F for approximately 15 minutes.

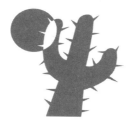

CHRISTINA'S MARGARITAS

Version 1 may cause brain freeze.
Version 2 is good after playing on a hot day.

YIELD: 1 SERVING PER OUNCE OF TEQUILA

3 measures margarita mix,
such as Jose Cuervo

1 measure Triple Sec

1 measure tequila

Coarse salt (optional)

Lemon or lime (optional)

Version 1

1. Put all of the ingredients into a blender, then fill with ice and blend. You should have equal parts liquid and ice in the blender.

2. Salt the rim of each margarita glass by moistening the rim with a cut of lemon, lime, or leftover margarita mix, and then dip the rim into a plate of salt.

3. Pour and enjoy.

Version 2

1. Put all of the ingredients into a sealed container. You can reuse the Jose Cuervo Margarita Mix bottle.

2. Put the container into the trunk of your car. (Don't place it next to your tennis bag, just in case it leaks!)

3. Drive to the tennis club and serve over ice cubes.

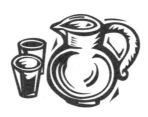

Tennis and Sisterfriends

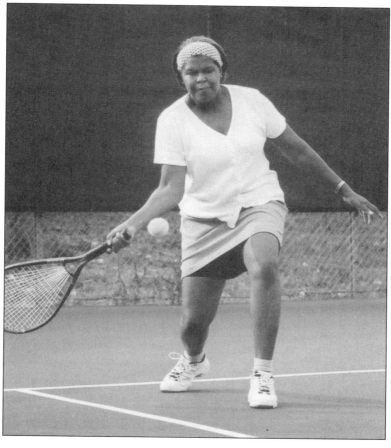

Don't forget to bend those knees!

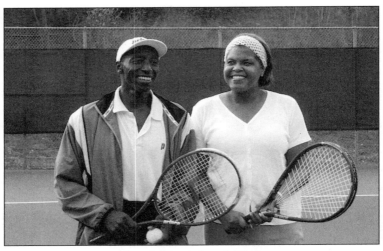

Coach Wendell and Alice.

There's no antiaging tonic more potent than time with the girls.

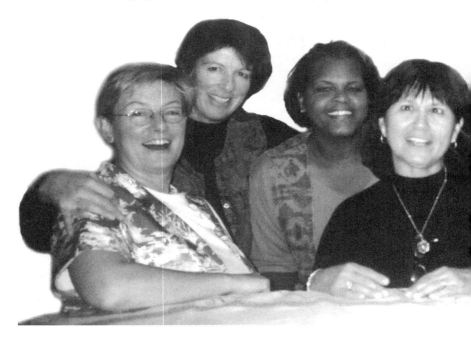

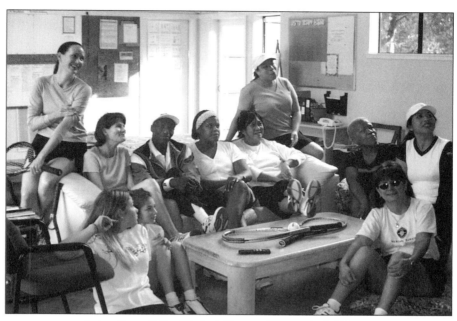

A meeting of the Chabot Canyon Women's 3.0 Team.

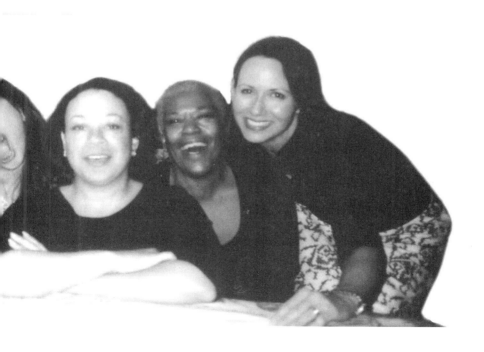

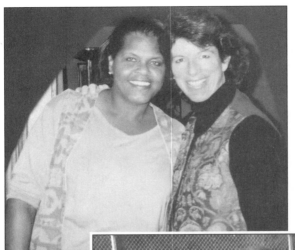

Alice and Coach Anne

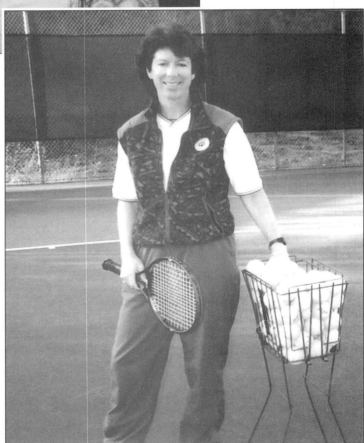

Coach Anne says, "Practice, practice, practice!"

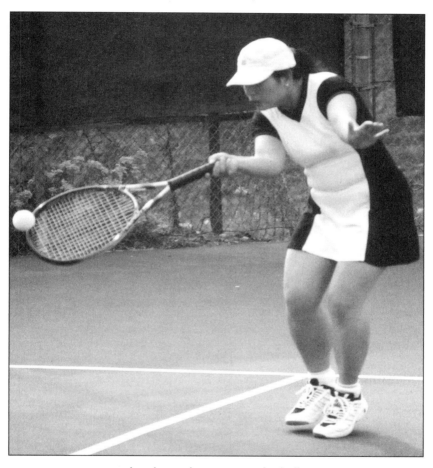

Lan keeps her eyes on the ball.

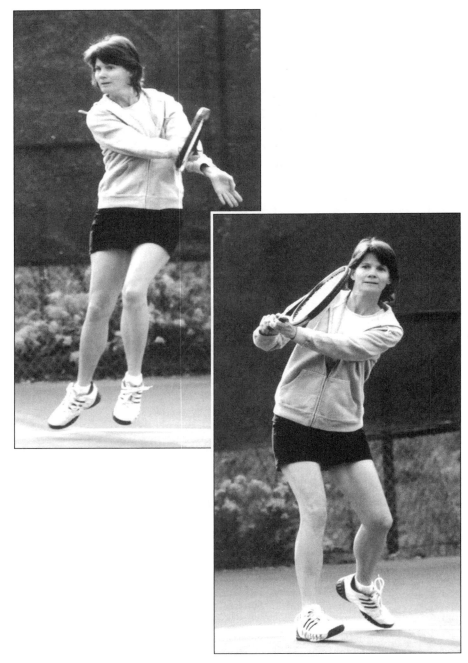

Linda keeps her feet moving.

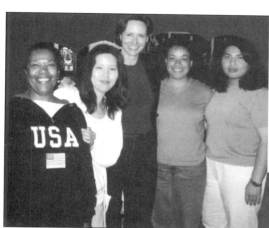

Phillis

Lauretta, Hitomi, Mary, Vanessa, and Lan (l to r)

Sisterfriends and food—the spices of life. Lan and Vanessa at the food table.

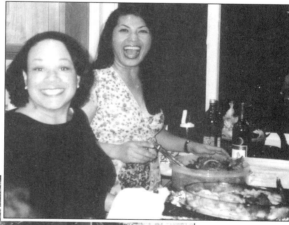

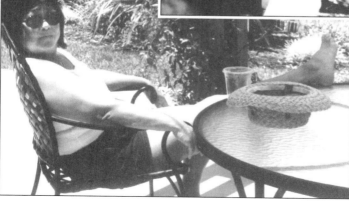

Jane kickin' it after a tough match.

About
the Author

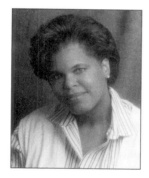

Alice Wilson-Fried is a proud postmenopausal woman, having survived five years of menopausal changes. She worked in public relations for the Delta Queen Steamboat Company in New Orleans before moving to northern California where she now resides with her husband. She is a writer, an avid tennis player, the mother of two, the stepmother of three, and grandmother of eight.